D1195847

SINGLE FIBRE
ELECTROMYOGRAPHY

by

Erik Stålberg and Jože V. Trontelj

The Mirvalle Press Limited
Old Woking, Surrey U.K. 1979

Distributed in the United States of America by Teca Corporation,
3 Campus Drive, Pleasantville, NY 10570 and by associated
companies and agencies throughout the world.

First Published 1979

British Library Cataloguing in Publication Data

Stålberg, Erik
  Single fibre electromyography.
  1. Electromyography
  I. Title   II. Trontelj, Jože V
  616.7′4′0754   RC77.5

ISBN 0–9506146–0–2

Produced by computer-controlled phototypesetting
using OCR input techniques and printed offset by
Unwin Brothers Limited
The Gresham Press, Old Woking, Surrey
A member of the Staples Printing Group

Dedicated to our wives and parents

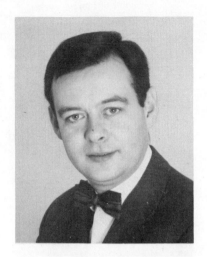

Erik Stålberg, born 1936, graduated from Medical School, Uppsala University 1963. He made his thesis on Propagation Velocity in Human Muscle Fibres 1966 at the Department of Pharmacology, Uppsala University. Since 1967 he has been working at the Department of Clinical Neurophysiology, University Hospital, Uppsala where he now is Associate Professor and head of the neuromuscular unit. He has together with Dr. J. Ekstedt developed the technique for Single Fibre Electromyography and has then introduced the method as a tool for research and routine in clinical neurophysiology.

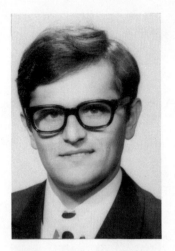

Jože V. Trontelj was born in 1939 in Yugoslavia. He is an Associate Professor of Neurology at the Medical Faculty, University of Ljubljana, and is working at the Institute of Clinical Neurophysiology, University Medical Center of Ljubljana.

He has been collaborating with Dr. Stålberg since 1967. His special interest is in human reflexology, where he introduced the technique of SFEMG, and in neuromuscular disorders. For his research he received the Award of the Boris Kidrič Fund in 1974.

PREFACE

Electromyography has become an invaluable tool for the study of the normal and the disordered motor system in man and animals. Its established role in neurophysiological research and clinical diagnosis has broadened, and it now also finds application in such diverse fields as ergonometry, the detection of intoxication by potentially harmful substances and the development of aids to rehabilitation. Increasing demands upon the electromyographer have been met by the refinement of existing techniques and the development of new ones, and this book gives an account of one such new approach, known as Single Fibre Electromyography (SFEMG).

It started when Dr. Jan Ekstedt and I became interested in measuring muscle fatigue. After a variety of recording methods had failed to meet our requirements, we were inspired by the multi-electrode of Buchthal, Rosenfalck and Guld to build a similar electrode with smaller recording surfaces. When, after what seemed a quite extravagant effort, we could be sure that the action potentials picked up by this electrode were indeed derived from single muscle fibres, our team work was presented in two theses, one on the jitter phenomenon and the other on muscle fibre action potential propagation velocity.

Collaboration with Dr. Jože Trontelj began in 1967 when he came to my laboratory and introduced the technique in Ljubljana.

Theoretical and technical considerations can be daunting, and our belief that SFEMG can enrich the repertoire of the clinical neurophysiologist has led us to adapt and simplify the method so that with patience, a little extra training and only minor modification of conventional equipment it can take its place in day-to-day diagnostic work.

The purpose of this book is to bring together, in the form of a general review rather than an exhaustive account of every study, the results of work with the single fibre needle electrode carried out in this and other laboratories over the past fifteen years. It seemed that a time had come when the knowledge gained might usefully be assembled for the information and guidance of present and prospective workers in the field, with some of whom the authors had the benefit and pleasure of discussion at an informal meeting in Uppsala in February 1977. Those present on that occasion were:

Lars Antoni, Uppsala, Sweden
John Ballantyne, Glasgow, Scotland
Sigge Blom, Umeå, Sweden
Poul Christensen, Skovlunde, Denmark
John W. Crayton, Chicago, Ill., U.S.A.
Jan Ekstedt, Umeå, Sweden
Robin Garnett, London, England
Isak Gath, Haifa, Israel
Domenico De Grandis, Verona, Italy
Stig Hansen, Glasgow, Scotland

Michael Hayward, Liverpool, England
Karl-Gösta Henriksson, Linkoping, Sweden
Per Hilton-Brown, Uppsala, Sweden
Evert Knutsson, Stockholm, Sweden
Lars Lindström, Göteborg, Sweden
Gösta Lovén, Uppsala, Sweden
Corrado Mezzini, Venice, Italy
Maria Teresa Niewiadomska-Wolska, Warsaw, Poland
Hiroshi Nishitani, Osaka, Japan
Peter Payan, London, England
Hans Schiller, Zurich, Switzerland
Martin S. Schwartz, London, England
Peter Styles, Old Woking, England
Michael Swash, London, England
Barbara Thiele, Berlin, Germany
Jean Vauthier, Brussels, Belgium
David B. Vodušek, Ljubljana, Yugoslavia
Janez Zidar, Ljubljana, Yugoslavia

It is hoped that this book may not only encourage the wider use of SFEMG in clinical and research studies, but also promote understanding of the findings of conventional electromyography, to which SFEMG is conceived as complementary and with which it does not compete.

September 1977   Erik Stålberg

ACKNOWLEDGEMENTS

We should like to thank Dr. Peter Payan for correcting the manuscript and for numerous valuable suggestions, and Dr. Robin Willison for his constructive criticism.

We are indebted to the many colleagues and collaborators who have contributed their technical and professional skills and help over the years of gathering experience with single fibre EMG. The following engineers deserve special mention for the merit they have shown in developing equipment and computer systems: Gösta Lovén, Janez Trontelj D.Sc., Lars Antoni and Marjan Mihelin M.Sc. We would also thank Annika Alsterlind, Charlotte Colliander, Siv Ehrnst, Miloš Kogej, Kerstin Mattson, Blaž Konec-Pinki, Alasdair McKinnon, Dr. David B. Vodušek, Dr. Janez Zidar and Matej Župančič.

To all our patients, and to the volunteers who participated in the investigations, we express our thanks.

The research has been supported for many years by the Swedish Medical Research Council and the Boris Kidrič Fund of Slovenia. Contributions have also been received from the Bob and Vivian Smith Foundation of Houston and the Child Care Council of Slovenia.

We would like to thank the Editors and Journals for the permission to use previously published figures according to the following:

Acta Anaesth. Scand.	fig: 55, 57
Annals of N.Y. Acad. Sci.	fig: 72, 73, 74, 75
Brain Research	fig: 95
Computer Programs in Biomedicine	fig: 3
Structure and Function of Normal and Diseased Muscle and Peripheral Nerve Polish Medical Publishers, Warsaw	fig: 30
Excerpta Medica, L.P. Rowland, Elsevier	fig: 43, 49, 81, 82 85, 86, 87
J. Neurol. Neurosurg. Psychiat.	fig: 15, 16, 29, 30, 35, 37, 79, 90, 93, 95
J. Neurol. Sci.	fig: 52, 53, 68, 69
New Developments in Electromyography and Clinical Neurophysiology, J.E. Desmedt, Karger, Basel	fig: 1, 44, 91, 94
The Motor System–Neurophysiology and Muscle Mechanisms, M. Shahani	fig: 70
Urologia Internationalis, Karger, Basel	fig: 97
Zdravstveni vestnik, Ljubljana	fig: 72

INTRODUCTORY NOTE

It is hoped that the cross-referencing provided will enable the book to be used as a manual.

An atlas of SFEMF recordings (to which reference is not made in the text) is included in order to help the reader to recognise some common artefacts and to gain some idea of what is typical of normal muscle and certain pathological states. Amplitude calibration has usually been omitted since, being extremely sensitive to electrode position, the amplitude of the action potential is not very useful in routine work. In illustrations with multiple traces, time sequence is upwards on recordings with a white background and downwards on recordings with a dark background unless otherwise indicated.

The references are arranged as follows: in the text the authors' own papers on SFEMG are referred to as numbers above the line, all other papers being referred to in the usual way. The latter are also represented in the Author index. The list of References at the end of the work is divided into SFEMG References (numbered) and General References (unnumbered).

TABLE OF CONTENTS

THE MOTOR UNIT

We may begin by considering briefly those basic morphological and physiological data which are pertinent to SFEMG studies.

The estimated number of muscle fibres belonging to a single motor unit varies from 9 in extraocular muscle to as many as 1900 in gastrocnemius (Feinstein, Lindegård, Nyman and Wohlfart, 1955). A neurophysiological technique (McComas, Fawcett, Campbell and Sica, 1971) suggests that the mean number of motor units is about 200 for extensor digitorum brevis muscle (McComas et al., 1971; Ballantyne and Hansen, 1974) and about 250-340 in the thenar muscles (McComas, 1977; Brown, 1972). All muscle fibres in a given unit are considered to have the same histochemical and mechanical characteristics, which are determined by the type of innervation. Thus, a slow muscle acquires the characteristics of a fast muscle when the nerve to a normally fast muscle is transplanted into it. In human voluntary muscle two main types of motor units (type I and type II) occur within one and the same muscle in varying, but often similar, proportions. A scattered anatomical arrangement of the muscle fibres belonging to a given motor unit has been demonstrated electrophysiologically in man (Ekstedt, 1964; Stålberg and Ekstedt, 1973; Stålberg, Schiller and Schwartz, 1975) and histochemically in animals (Kugelberg and Edström, 1968; Brandstater and Lambert, 1969; Doyle and Mayer, 1969, Fig. 1). Furthermore low and high threshold motor units have been shown to have important differences in their histochemical (Warmolts and Engel, 1973) and mechanical characteristics (Edström and Kugelberg, 1968; Milner-Brown, Stein and Yemm, 1973a; Burke, Tsairis, Levine, Zajac and Engel, 1973). Dependence of activation threshold upon neurone size and axon diameter has been suggested by Henneman, Somjen and Carpenter (1965), and correlation between activation threshold and axon diameter has been noted in man (Freund, Dietz, Wita and Kapp, 1973). Correlation was also found between the activation threshold and the size of the motor unit in man (Milner-Brown, Stein and Yemm, 1973a). The firing pattern and recruitment order of motor units during voluntary contraction have been studied by many authors, some showing two types of pattern corresponding to tonic and phasic motor units (Tokizane and Shimazu, 1964), others reporting a continuum of the firing characteristics from irregular to regular innervation rates (Petajan and Philip, 1969; Milner-Brown, Stein and Yemm, 1973b, c). The recruitment order of voluntarily activated motor units varies little with different manoeuvres, but can be changed within certain limits (Grimby and Hannerz, 1968 and 1975).

Many of the methods used in the above-mentioned research are inapplicable to man, in whom the most commonly used method for the study of the disordered motor unit is concentric needle EMG, introduced by Adrian and Bronk in 1929.

1

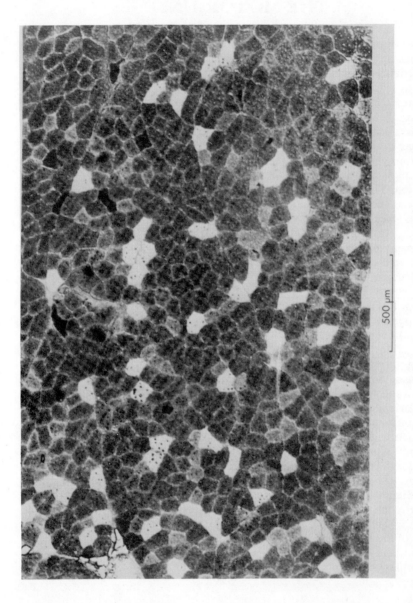

500 µm

Fig. 1   Scattered arrangement of muscle fibres in a motor unit. Muscle fibres belonging to one motor unit in the rat tibialis anterior muscle have been depleted of glycogen by prolonged electrical stimulation of its axon. They appear pale in glycogen staining (From Kugelberg, 1973).

CONCENTRIC NEEDLE ELECTROMYOGRAPHY (CNEMG)

It is important to establish at the outset that SFEMG is not merely a miniature form of CNEMG: it focuses on different motor unit characteristics. The two techniques are therefore complementary, and the results of each may illumine those of the other. The following discussion of CNEMG is intended only as a background against which to consider the SFEMG method, and for a detailed description the reader is referred to established texts (e.g. Licht, 1971; Goodgold and Eberstein, 1972; Hopf and Struppler, 1974; Ludin, 1976; Lenman and Ritchie, 1977).

The so called motor unit potential (MUP) recorded with a concentric needle electrode is generated by the muscle fibres from one motor unit. The amplitude and shape of the MUP is determined by the number of muscle fibres within the recording area of the electrode, their spatial arrangement in relation to the electrode and the temporal relationship between the individual single muscle fibre action potentials. One and the same motor unit can thus give rise to many different MUPs depending on the position of the electrode. Only those muscle fibres lying within about one millimetre of the leading-off surface of the electrode (typically less than 20; Thiele and Boehle, 1975) contribute to the spike of the MUP. More distant fibres are responsible for the slower components of the potential owing to a low-pass filter effect of muscle tissue on volume conduction.

The MUP is characterised by its appearance and its firing pattern. It is usual to specify: (1) duration (2) configuration, or number of phases (3) amplitude and (4) variability in shape at consecutive discharges. Sometimes the territory of the motor unit is also measured. In addition to the electrode position and its electrical characteristics, these parameters depend on the number and size of the muscle fibres, the conduction time in terminal nerve branches and muscle fibres and the location of the motor end-plates relative to the electrode. The varying contributions of these factors mean that the characteristics of many MUPs must be averaged and compared to normal values, which themselves depend on temperature, age and the muscle under consideration. Individual MUPs can be measured only during slight voluntary contraction, when they are visually separable from one another. Stronger or maximal effort results in an interference pattern of varying density and amplitude depending upon the number of motor units activated, their firing rate and the individual properties of the MUPs.

The range of normal values is often broad, and it may be difficult to be certain whether a given finding is pathological or not. Quantitative measurements of different kinds improve the accuracy of the analysis, but are not infallible. Nevertheless, certain clear-cut pictures emerge, such as the drop-out of individual muscle fibres in myopathies and of whole motor units in neuropathies, the grouping and increased number of fibres within motor units in reinnervation, and the low firing rate in upper motor neurone lesions.

More detailed consideration shows that in primary myopathies MUPs are typically polyphasic, of low amplitude and short duration — although exceptionally long potentials are sometimes encountered in Duchenne's dystrophy. The interference pattern is full but often of low amplitude. Similar "myopathic" changes may occur in acute peripheral denervation, early reinnervation and in myasthenia gravis. In an acute neuronal lesion few motor units may be recruited but MUPs are normal. With reinnervation the potentials become polyphasic and initially of unstable form. Long-duration, stable potentials, usually of large amplitude, occur in chronic partial denervation. When the neurogenic disorder is progressive the long polyphasic potentials become variable in form. An often neglected factor is the effect upon volume conduction, and hence the properties of the MUP, of muscle fibrosis and fatty replacement. These changes may theoretically restrict volume conduction, causing an increase in the recorded amplitude of individual muscle fibre potentials and a consequently increased MUP amplitude. When the process is more pronounced, successively more muscle fibres will be "shielded" from the recording position, resulting in reduced MUP amplitude. In all the conditions mentioned, spontaneous activity of various kinds may occur: fibrillation potentials, and positive sharp waves, high-frequency repetitive discharges of single or many muscle fibres, and spontaneously occurring potentials, similar to MUPs, in conjunction with visible muscle fasciculation.

The CNEMG electrode provides an overall picture of the structure and function of the individual motor unit and of the concerted action of the units employed at a given effort. Information concerning the individual elements generating the MUP is not directly obtained by this means, however, and it is in the attempt to study the physiology of the motor unit at this level that single muscle fibre EMG has proved valuable.

SELECTIVE RECORDING

BACKGROUND

The resting membrane potential of the muscle fibre is about 80 mV, inside negative. A nerve impulse arriving at the motor end-plate, which lies somewhere near the middle of the length of the muscle fibre, releases acetylcholine which initiates membrane depolarisation. From the end-plate region a wave of depolarisation is propagated continuously along the muscle fibre towards its ends, and the moving electrical field can be recorded outside the muscle fibre as an action potential.

Although in theory the maximum action potential decreases exponentially with increasing recording distance,[22,23,24] in practice there are always distortions. The electrical field is shunted by the metallic leading-off surface, and an average value of the isopotential lines crossing the electrode surface is recorded (Fig. 2). Due to the smaller radius of the isopotential lines and the higher gradient of the electrical field close to the muscle fibre distortion is most pronounced at small recording distances, when the amplitude will be less than estimated for a theoretical recording with a point-shaped electrode; with longer fibre-electrode distances distortion is less marked. This shunting effect is pronounced when, as in the case of the commonly used concentric needle electrode, the leading-off surface of 150×580 μm is large in relation to the muscle fibre which has a diameter of 25–100 μm. Thus, while the closest muscle fibres naturally have the highest recorded amplitude, the difference between the amplitude of potentials deriving from near and from distant fibres is much less than might be expected.

SMALL ELECTRODES

From the foregoing considerations it follows that a more selective recording may be expected from a small electrode, which should increase the ratio in amplitude between potentials recorded from adjacent and distant muscle fibres. In practice the near muscle fibres give rise to higher action potentials than are recorded with a conventional concentric needle electrode and, with appropriate amplifier gain, action potentials from distant fibres are very small or not even discernible. The selectivity is enhanced by the fact that such a small leading-off surface is likely to be near fewer muscle fibres belonging to one unit than would be the concentric needle electrode surface. An electrode diameter of 25–30 μm has been shown to be optimal[16] (Fig. 3). This is smaller than the average normal muscle fibre diameter and causes only minimal shunting of the action potential, as is evident from comparison with that theoretically obtained for the point-shaped electrode. With a smaller leading-off surface the electrode impedance would increase, which might introduce problems with input amplifier circuits without offering any practical recording advantage.

5

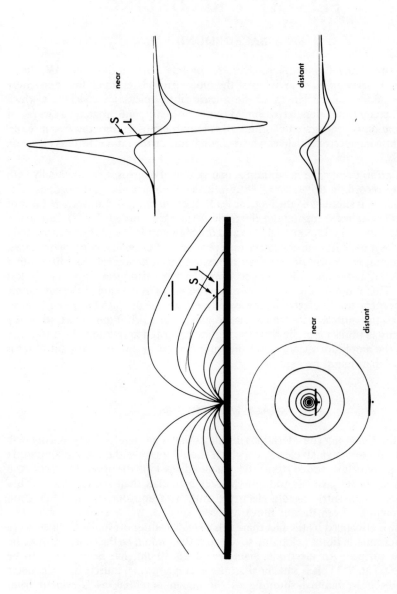

Fig. 2   The electrical field around a muscle fibre recorded with a small (S) and a large (L) electrode surface. The large electrode shunts the isopotential lines at short fibre-electrode distances, but less so at longer distances. Thus at a short distance, the large electrode records lower amplitude of the action potential than the small electrode.

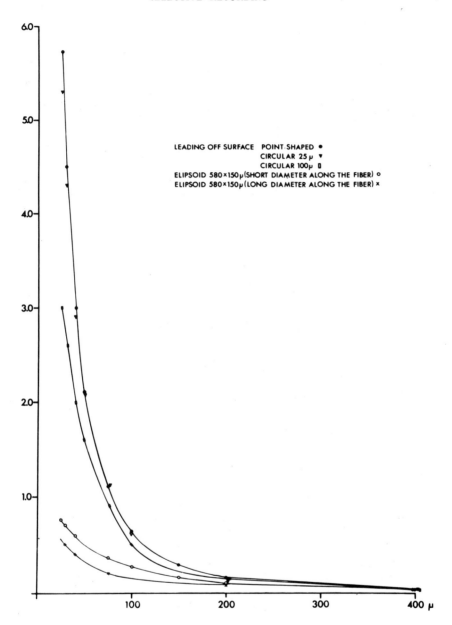

LEADING OFF SURFACE POINT-SHAPED •
CIRCULAR 25 μ ▾
CIRCULAR 100μ ▯
ELIPSOID 580×150μ (SHORT DIAMETER ALONG THE FIBER) ○
ELIPSOID 580×150μ (LONG DIAMETER ALONG THE FIBER) ×

Fig. 3   The amplitude (ordinate in arbitrary units) versus recording distance for simulated action potentials recorded with different types of leading-off surfaces. Note the low amplitude obtained with large electrodes for short electrode-fibre distance. Recording conditions for point-shaped and 25 μm electrode are similar (From Ekstedt and Stålberg, 1973a).

Wire Electrodes

The simplest way to obtain an electrode with a small recording area is to record from the bare tip of a thin insulated wire inserted into the muscle. The wire diameters most commonly used are 50–100 μm. The wire is introduced by means of an injection cannula which is then withdrawn. An even smaller recording surface can be obtained by making a small hole in the insulation coat by means of a spark. The size of the hole can be of the order of 10–20 μm (Hannerz, 1975). With such small surfaces the shape of single fibre potentials is liable to distortion but selectivity is high, owing to the filter characteristics of the electrode (high pass filter). The size and impedance of this kind of electrode are inevitably very difficult to standardise, and quantitative studies such as the analysis of action potential shape and the estimation of fibre density are not possible. Furthermore, it is impossible to make the necessary fine adjustments of the recording position.

Needle Electrodes

An electrode with more consistent characteristics is obtained by inserting the wire into a cannula, exposing its end at a side port a few millimetres behind the tip (Fig. 4) and grinding it flush with the surrounding epoxy resin. Electrodes with up to 14 such leading-off surfaces have been constructed.[8] This insulating area provides the so called *wall effect*, which will increase the recorded amplitude by a factor of 2. This type of electrode is used for the studies presented in this book and will be called the *SFEMG electrode*.

"BIPOLAR" RECORDING

The selectivity of the EMG recording can be increased even beyond that obtained by using a small recording surface. One way is to use differential recording between two small electrodes with a short interelectrode distance, i.e. so-called "bipolar" recording, in which the net signal represents the difference between the signals recorded at each of the two electrodes. Action potentials from fibres equidistant from the two electrodes will be cancelled and thus the uptake area will be restricted and the recording very selective (Fig. 5). The optimal position is with one of the two recording surfaces close to the muscle fibre studied, and with the other (reference) surface at a right angle to the fibre. The interelectrode distance should not exceed 200 μm. If the interelectrode distance is too small the recorded action potential will decrease significantly. If the interelectrode distance is too large, the electrodes will be picking up from two independent sources and no common activity will be cancelled. The action potentials picked up with the so called reference electrode will appear with reversed polarity and can thus be identified.

FILTER

When the action potential is volume-conducted through the muscle tissue the different frequency components of the signal are attenuated to different degrees. The tissue is similar to a low pass filter in that the action potential loses its high frequency components relatively faster than its low frequency components. In other

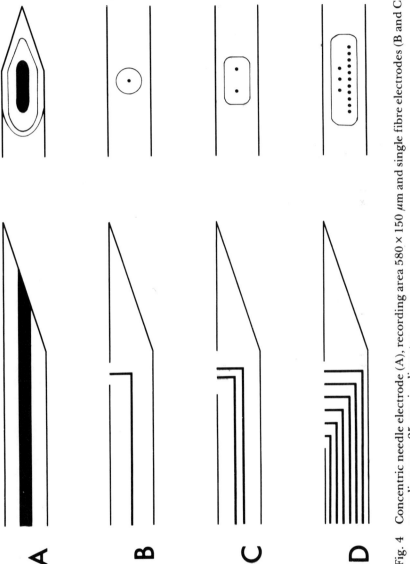

Fig. 4 Concentric needle electrode (A), recording area 580 × 150 μm and single fibre electrodes (B and C), recording area 25 μm in diameter.

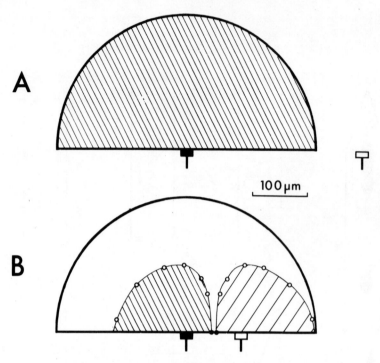

Fig. 5   Recording with different reference electrodes.
A. "Monopolar" recording with a reference electrode outside the muscle. The hatched semi-circle delineates the recording area within which the action potential is recorded with 5% (at the border) to 100% of its amplitude (close to the electrode).
B. "Bipolar" recording with inter-electrode distance of 100 μm. The recording area is markedly reduced. The action potentials recorded with the reference surface within the lightly hatched area appear with reversed polarity.
The diagram is based on data taken from fig 3.

words, the action potentials recorded from distant muscle fibres contain a larger proportion of low frequency components than those from adjacent muscle fibres. This fact can be exploited to reduce the interference from distant muscle fibres and thus increase the selectivity of the recording. By reducing the low frequency response of the amplifier, the amplitude of distant fibre action potentials is attenuated more than that of an adjacent muscle fibre. With the high pass filter at 100 Hz (roll off = 12 dB per octave) only slight improvement is obtained, except for the reduction in slow movement artefacts, but at 500 Hz a significant reduction of background activity is achieved. The amplitude of the action potentials from fibres close to the electrode is reduced by less than 10%, whereas distant fibre action potentials are reduced more substantially. At more extreme filter settings of 1000–5000 Hz the recorded action potentials become gradually reduced to the first derivative of the original signal. The amplitude is then correlated to the rise time of the original action potential[21] (Fig.6).

By combining small electrode, bipolar derivation and high pass filtering, a single fibre potential can sometimes be followed undisturbed by other active muscle fibres at up to 50–75 per cent of maximal muscle force. Similar conclusions concerning selective recording were presented, for example, by Andreassen and Rosenfalck (1977). With increasing selectivity the recording position becomes gradually more critical.

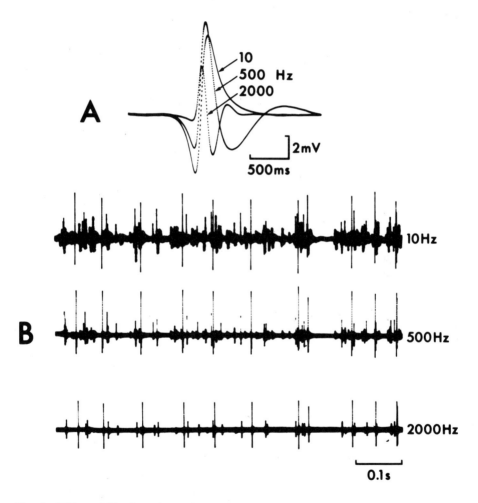

Fig. 6   Effect of filtering. A, on the shape and amplitude of the single fibre action potential. B, on the background activity.

THE SINGLE MUSCLE FIBRE
ACTION POTENTIAL

THE SHAPE

The single fibre action potential recorded with the SFEMG electrode in optimal position is a biphasic spike with a positive-negative going fast deflection having a rise time of 75–200 μs (depending on the distance between muscle fibre and recording electrode and on the propagation velocity of the muscle fibre) and a total duration of about one millisecond[7] (Fig. 6). The shape is constant at consecutive discharges when the recording system has a resolution of 5–10 μs. The amplitude, positively correlated to the diameter of the muscle fibre, is extremely dependent on the recording distance. The radial attenuation of the action potential amplitude is exponential.[23]

When the position of the electrode is adjusted so as to give a maximal single fibre action potential the recorded amplitude is usually between 1 and 7 mV with occasional values of 15–20 mV. Most of the spectral energy is concentrated between 100 Hz and 10 KHz, with a peak value at 1.61 ± 0.30 KHz and -3 dB points at 0.91 ± 0.19 KHz and 2.41 ± 0.53 KHz (Fig. 7)[21] When the recording distance is increased, the power spectrum of the action potential is changed, and this has been further studied with a multi-electrode technique.

VOLUME CONDUCTION

Many studies on the volume conduction of the extracellular muscle fibre action potential have been based on mathematical models (Rosenfalck, 1969), in which assumptions are made as to homogeneity (homogeneous: all parts have the same conductivity) and isotropy (isotropy: the conductivity is the same in all directions) in order to simplify calculation of the radial decline of the extracellular action potential. Many of these models are based on data obtained from in vitro measurements in artifically simplified conditions (Håkansson, 1956, 1957).

The radial decline of the extracellular muscle fibre action potential has been investigated in situ[23,24] in order to obtain information about the volume conduction characteristics of muscle tissue and also about the homogeneity and isotropy of the muscle.

A multi-electrode was used in which 14 leading-off surfaces each 25 μm in diameter were arranged in two rows of 12 and 2 (a modification of the electrode shown in Fig. 4D). The average distance between adjacent leading-off surfaces was 40 μm. The electrode was inserted perpendicularly to the fibre direction, and the action potential from one muscle fibre was recorded from all electrodes. The analysis was mainly from four electrodes, i.e. between the one closest to the fibre and each of three at respective distances of 79, 152 and 251 μm. Thus three muscle sections of different length were studied.

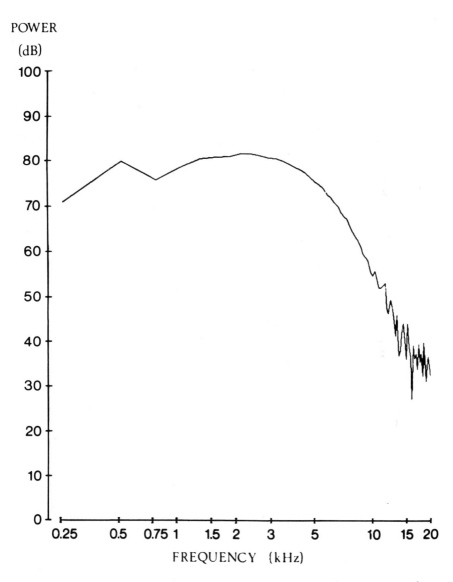

Fig. 7 Power spectrum of a single muscle fibre action potential. Ordinate: Power spectrum normalized with a total mean square value. Abscissa: Frequency.

Fourier transformation of the action potential was carried out by a standard Fast Fourier Transform routine. The transfer function of a section of muscle tissue was calculated from the Fourier transform of the input and output of this section, i.e. from the action potentials recorded at the two neighbouring electrodes.

Single tissue section could be simulated by one RC section having the following transfer function $|T(j\omega)|$

$$|T(j\omega)| = \frac{K}{\sqrt{1 + (\omega\tau)^2}}$$

where K is the gain factor, ω the angular frequency and τ the time constant. The average gain factor K was 0.51 and the average time constant, calculated at the −3 db point was found to be 69 μs.

The average attentuation of the sinusoidal components of the action potential for a distance of 76 μm was calculated from $T(j\omega)$. For the frequencies 240 Hz, 1900 Hz and 3800 Hz the attenuation was −5.2 dB, −7.4 dB and −10.9 dB respectively. The distance at which a 3800 Hz sinusoidal component declines to one tenth of its maximal amplitude is roughly half that for 240 Hz. The results of these measurements, showing an exponential decline of the sinusoidal components of the action potential *in situ*, are qualitatively in agreement with theoretical considerations describing the attenuation of the electrical field in dissipative media (Adler, Chu and Fano, 1960). Quantitatively the present study shows a greater attenuation with distance of the sinusoidal components of the action potential than has previously been described. The effect is most conspicuous for lower frequencies, whereas for frequencies higher than 3000 Hz our results are similar to those of Rosenfalck (1969) calculated for anisotropic conditions. These studies are in agreement with our previous investigations[16] and show a greater radial decline of the overall signal than reported by Krnjević and Miledi (1958) and by Buchthal, Guld and Rosenfalck (1957).

One source of the discrepancy between this and other studies might be the type of electrode used in the different investigations. The spectral content of the recorded signal is determined not only by the source but also by the filter function of the needle electrodes. Previous investigators have used larger electrodes which distort the signal more than those used in this study. Another possible reason for discrepancy, particularly in the greater radial attenuation of the slow frequencies of the action potential, may be a greater anisotropy of the muscle investigated than is assumed in some mathematical models. This effect has been predicted by Lindström (1973) in his mathematical model.

EQUIPMENT

ELECTRODES

SFEMG Electrodes

All SFEMG electrodes are built according to the same general principle, with a steel cannula 0.5 to 0.6 mm in diameter inside which 1 to 14 insulated platinum or silver wires are placed and taken out at a side port one to three millimetres behind the tip (Fig. 4).[8] The port is in the side opposite to the bevelled surface in order to avoid recording from mechanically compressed or damaged muscle fibres. The electrodes are embedded in epoxy resin throughout the entire cannula. Each of the wires is connected to one pin in the plug.

In the multi-electrode study the patient is grounded via the electrode shaft. The reference electrode is a subcutaneous needle electrode, or the multi-electrode shaft. In this type of electrode there is an interelectrode capacitance of 8–10 $\mu \mu$F for the different electrode combinations, further increased by 5–10 $\mu \mu$F in the input cable of the amplifiers. This gives rise to a capacitative crosstalk of the signals between the different leads proportional to the rate of rise of the voltage differences. The crosstalk signal may be of the order of 4% but can be considerably reduced by using one of the electrode surfaces in the multi-electrode as reference. Approximately similar crosstalk signals are then fed to both inputs of the amplifier and thereby cancelled. This is possible when the reference electrode is known not to pick up any significant activity from the muscle fibre under study.

When recording with single or double surface electrodes the cannula is used as a reference electrode and is connected to the amplifier input. In this situation the patient is grounded with a cutaneous pad electrode placed not far away over an electrically fairly silent area, usually an antagonistic muscle. In the multi-electrode or in the double-surface electrode bipolar recordings between two electrode surfaces can be made when the greatest possible selectivity is required.

For jitter measurements, fibre density measurements, firing pattern studies and reflex studies an electrode with one recording surface is enough. Multi-electrode studies are used for measurements of muscle fibre propagation velocity, for volume conduction studies, and for detailed studies of motor unit arrangement. The electrode surfaces are arranged geometrically in different ways in the port according to specific need.

The Macro-Micro Electrode

In some studies it has been of interest to record simultaneously from a single muscle fibre and from many muscle fibres in the same motor unit by means of a combined electrode with a small and a large electrode surface. This is most easily obtained with a minor modification of the connections in the side port SFEMG electrode, the recording being made both from the small side port leading-off surface and a big leading-off surface represented by the cannula, perhaps restricted by insulation except for the tip region; another indifferent electrode must then be used. However, it is usually of greater interest to compare SFEMG recordings with the motor unit potential as obtained with a concentric needle electrode. Hence the "macro" surface should resemble that of an ordinary concentric EMG needle. For this purpose some different electrode types have been constructed. The two electrodes have been placed in the tip of the cannula, the small electrode close to the surface being identical to that in the concentric needle electrode. In this construction the 25 μm wire is also cut obliquely and will have an oval shape measuring 25 × 100 μm with the standard tip angle of 15°. In another construction the small electrode has been placed in a side port and the larger in the tip but now the distance between the recording sites is usually too large to allow reasonable comparison between the two recordings. Different electrodes have also been constructed with both the small and the large surface in the side port. The large surface is made to have the same dimensions as in the tip of the concentric needle electrode, about 150 × 580 μm. Different spatial relationships between the two leading-off surfaces have been tested; the most convenient seems to be the one with the small electrode 50–100 μm from the large electrode at the level of its centre region (Fig. 8). This electrode can be used for recording the conventional motor unit action potential simultaneously with the action potential from a single muscle fibre. Action potentials of muscle fibres most closely adjacent to both recording electrodes have a small time lag between the two recordings corresponding to the propagation time over the interelectrode gap and this has to be taken into consideration when time comparisons are made.

The Injection Electrode

This electrode consists of two platinum leading-off surfaces in the side port of the cannula on either side of the mouth of a glass capillary with an inner diameter of 150 μm. Microinjections can be made close to the muscle fibre from which the recording is made.

Marking Electrode

Correlation between electromyographical phenomena and the histological picture of the exact site from which the recording is made is of considerable interest. For this purpose an electrode has been constructed which allows marking of the site of recording. On either side of the recording surface and close to it there is a silver surface about 25 μm in diameter. A weak alternating current is passed through to deposit some silver in the tissue.

SFEMG with Concentric Needle Electrode

It is occasionally possible to record single fibre action potentials with an ordinary concentric needle electrode, particularly if the low frequencies of the signal below 500–1000 Hz be cut; in this way both increased jitter and impulse blocking can be detected (e.g. Borenstein and Desmedt, 1975). Such filtering may, however, cause a spike component to resemble a true single fibre action potential whereas it is actually composed of more than one. When this happens the jitter may be underestimated due to a summation effect, so that the concentric needle electrode is unsuitable for the detection of mild jitter abnormality. It is clearly also unsuitable for accurate fibre density measurements.

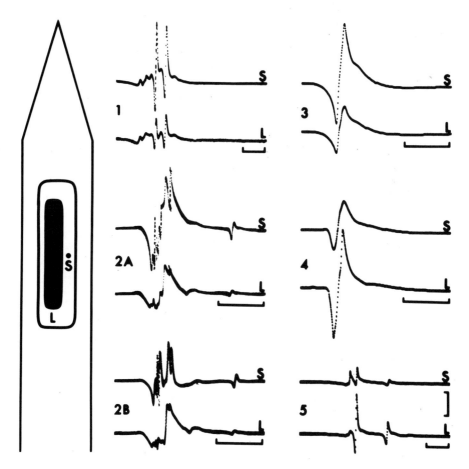

Fig. 8 Macro-micro electrode with a small (S) and a large (L) surface. 1. Typical
recording. Spike components recorded by small surface have larger
amplitude. 2. Another recording with the same filter settings (3.2 Hz–16
kHz) for both amplifiers (A) and with low frequency response for the small
electrode set up to 500 Hz (B). 3. Optimal position for the small electrode. 4.
Another motor unit. Position of small surface is not adjusted optimally for
the nearest fibres. 5. Similar to 4. Two fibres are passing the electrode, but
are not close to the small surface. Calibrations 2 ms and 1 mV.

Treatment of the Electrode

The tip: A hook on the electrode tip, caused, for example, by having touched bone, will damage the muscle fibres closest to the electrode, which are the fibres from which the optimal recordings are to be made. As a result, an increased proportion of false double potentials may be recorded (page 59). In addition, damaged fibres may become silent. Whenever a hook is suspected (felt as a resistance on inserting needle into muscle) the tip must be checked either with a piece of cotton wool moved along the needle axis toward the tip or under the microscope. Regrinding with stone paper or an Arkansas stone should then be done. The tip may be made extra sharp and resistant by grinding it to a plough shape from the side of the needle which is 180° from the bevelled surface. The needle shaft should be kept smooth to avoid damage to and mechanical displacement of muscle fibres, though slight roughness of the shaft surface may help to maintain a desired position in the muscle.

The electrode surface: The insulating epoxy resin can sometimes, particularly when the electrode is new, change its volume slightly after autoclaving or sterilizing in boiling water. Even the slightest protrusion of this material can make recording difficult because the sliding of muscle fibres over the electrode is hindered and because the leading-off surface may be retracted. In these situations the side port must be smoothed off with stone paper, e.g. 600 silicon carbide. It is also possible to use a wooden stick for polishing the epoxy, recording surface and shaft. After a number of recording sessions (about five) the small leading-off surface may become polarised or deposits of material from the muscle may stick to it. When using platinum wire the electrode can be electrolytically treated by sending a current through it. The electrode is placed in a small bath of saline and the negative pole of a 4.5 V battery is connected via 0.1 Mohm resistor to the recording surface. The positive pole is connected to a metallic rod (an injection cannula) in the bath. The 10 to 20 μA current is passed through the electrodes for 10–20 seconds under microscopic control. This D.C. current produces small bubbles from the electrode surface which is in this way cleaned and its resistance reduced.[8]

Note: If silver electrodes are used, electrolytic treatment should never be performed or silver ions will simply be removed and the leading-off surface will disappear back into epoxy resin. Here the cleaning of the electrode surface should be effected with stone paper.

AMPLIFIERS

The electrode leading-off surface has relatively high electrical impedance, different for different metals in the wires. For platinum this is of the order of 100 Kohm at 1000 Hz, 1 mV. A high amplifier input resistance and a low input capacitance are therefore necessary to give a sufficiently high frequency response of the system to allow the single fibre action potentials to be recorded undistorted and to reduce crosstalk in the multi-electrode recordings. The input impedance of the amplifier should be of the order of 100 Mohm for the platinum electrodes.

In our equipment each leading-off surface is connected to its own pre-amplifier via an electrode cable 30 cm long. This is an impedance converter and has a gain of × 1 or

× 100. Each input lead is individually screened and the screen is driven by positive feedback from the particular pre-amplifier in order to reduce the input capacitance. All input leads, furthermore, have a common grounded screen. Other means of reducing the input capacitance are also available. For the multi-electrode recordings, mechanically or digitally operated electrode selectors work after the pre-amplifiers, i.e. in the low impedance circuits. These select active and reference electrodes for three independent amplifiers. With the electrode and the amplifier connected, the common mode rejection should be better than 200. The frequency response curve for the system should preferably be flat between 2 and 20,000 Hz (see below). No appreciable phase shift within the flat part of the frequency response curve can be accepted when action potential analysis is to be made.

The slow components picked up during the recording are often due to interfering activity from distant muscle fibres. This disturbing activity can be greatly reduced by setting the high-pass filters to 500 Hz; this will slightly change the shape of the single fibre action potential under study, which does not matter when measurements of propagation velocity, jitter and fibre density are to be made. When detailed studies of action potential shape are to be performed, the high-pass filter setting should be about 2 Hz.

Modern EMG equipment has amplifiers fulfilling the requirements described.

LOUDSPEAKER

Acoustical information is an essential part of almost any SFEMG study. This is particularly true when the investigator is looking for multiple potentials. The single fibre action potential has a clear high-pitched sound and the double potential a typical cracked echo-like sound, or the sound of castanets. An experienced investigator can detect blocking by ear, and even estimate the length of the interpotential interval and the degree of jitter. Because of this the final positioning of the needle can be achieved by sound better than by the picture on the screen. Sound may also indicate that there is an early component of low amplitude preceding a later triggering action potential. The same applies to late components when these are not seen on the screen of the oscilloscope owing to too high a sweep speed. For the patient, the loudspeaker is a form of feed-back which helps him to control the firing rate as well as to modify the degree of contraction to a desired level.

The quality of the loudspeaker supplied with the better EMG equipment is adequate, although a big extra loudspeaker is often an advantage. In multi-electrode studies, acoustical signals from two recording sites may be presented stereophonically.

RATE METER

In order to allow the patient to monitor the mean firing rate and degree of irregularity, a rate meter can be used. In our equipment a tachometer from a car is adjusted to a frequency range of 0–100 Hz. The gate pulse from the oscilloscope triggered by the action potential is fed to the tachometer. When the firing rate is to be studied, the patient is instructed to keep the rate as steady as possible. Short training prior to investigation enables most people to do this with a considerable degree of accuracy. These measurements are made when the firing pattern itself is studied, or when the effect of different mean frequency or varying interdischarge intervals is correlated to propagation velocity (page 74) or to neuromuscular jitter and blocking (page 124).

TAPE RECORDER

It is convenient to store the recording on magnetic tape for later analysis. A variety of tape recorders can be used, but they must fulfil certain minimum requirements, which vary according to the type of study.

Frequency Response

Single fibre action potentials have little spectral energy below 100 Hz and above 10 KHz, and this frequency range is covered by most of the better AM tape recorders. Some of the better FM tape recorders will give satisfactory reproduction when used at very high tape speed. The FM mode will also reduce the amplitude variation of the recorded signal, the flutter. When the shape of the action potential is studied a broad bandwidth is required, obtained for the lowest cost in AM tape recorders. For surface-recorded EMG signals with low-frequency components, FM tape recorders are necessary.

In many SFEMG applications interest is focused on time measurements in which action potentials are used as event markers. The desired accuracy of these measurements is of the order of 5 μs. Therefore the wow of the tape recorder should not exceed this value over time intervals of 0.5–4 ms. The flutter should also be low because it can change the triggering point on the potential slope and so artificially increase the measured jitter. To reduce the flutter the heads should be kept clean and the tape guides checked regularly.

Tape Recorder Test

Frequency response is tested in the same way as with amplifiers, using sine waves of varying frequencies. The *wow* is tested with repetitive double square pulses at intervals of 0.5–4 ms and the jitter is measured according to techniques given on page 43. The wow, measured as MCD between constant double square pulses with pulse intervals up to 4 ms, is usually 2–4 μs. This value does not usually have a significant influence on the recorded jitter except when the latter is less than 10 μs (see page 55). This variability is too large for detailed analysis of propagation time across the needle and its variability, which is of the order of 0.1–3 μs. In this case, measurements have to be done on-line. The *flutter* is seen as variation in the amplitude of high frequency (5 KHz) sine waves when using a low oscilloscope sweep speed.

For analysis of jitter, ordinary cassette tape recorders available at present may have an adequate frequency response but owing to mechanical instability in tape transport the wow introduces an unacceptable error. A high quality home tape recorder of reel type fulfils the frequency response demands.

For the analysis of action potential shape the lower frequency response limit and the flutter of an analogue reel tape recorder is apt to provide inaccurate data, and analysis should therefore be done on-line if possible, or the signal stored in digital form after on-line fast A/D conversion.

DISPLAY

Single fibre action potentials are usually displayed on an oscilloscope screen with a sweep speed between 2 and 0.1 ms/div., depending on the particular study. When measuring fibre density, firing pattern or extra-discharges the slower sweep speeds are used, but for the study of jitter or propagation velocity a higher sweep speed is more suitable. Some means of improving the display are as follows:

Delay Line

To obtain a stable recording the action potential should preferably be triggered on its fast positive-negative going deflection as close to the zero intersection point as possible. In doing so the initial part of the action potential is lost. This is overcome by the use of a delay line, analogue or digital, with at least 0.5 ms delay. The frequency response of the delay line, as well as introduced phase distortions, should be tested. Furthermore, analogue delay lines introduce a "ringing" after transients and fast components of an action potential, especially with longer delays. In extreme cases this may cause extra phases in the single fibre action potential.

Time Base

In order to analyse a component coming more than 2 ms after the trigger with the sweep speed commonly used, some special arrangement has to be made (Fig. 9). Many standard oscilloscopes have the option of *sweep magnification* (× 10) around the middle of the sweep. The component to be studied can in this way be expanded for display, though the triggering potential will be lost. In *dual beam-dual time base* oscilloscopes the second beam, with appropriate sweep speed, can be triggered on saw-tooth voltage of the first beam ("starts after delay interval"). The whole potential may then be displayed at a slow sweep speed on the first beam and the interesting part analysed on the second.

A special device with *dual sweep time* allows a slow sweep speed to change to a fast standard speed (e.g. 0.2 ms/div.) at an optional position along the sweep. The triggering potential is now seen with a lower time resolution. Another possibility is *"sweep compression"*, that is stopping or, better, markedly reducing the sweep speed at any position and for any chosen time and then continuing. In this way both triggering and late components can be displayed with high resolution.

This can also be accomplished by *retriggering* the fast sweep after a preset delay following the initial triggering potential, which involves the loss of a certain period of time between the two sweeps.

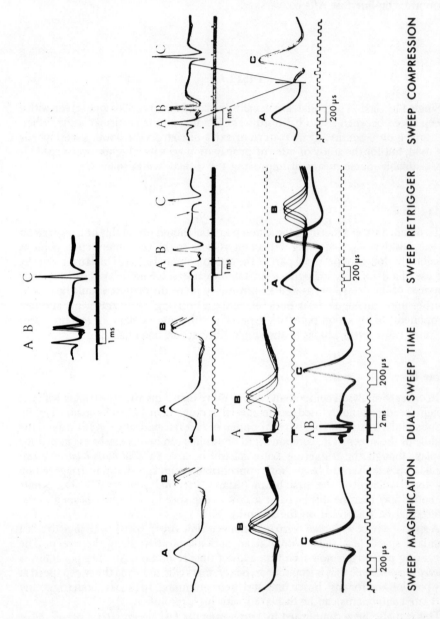

Fig. 9 Different possibilities of displaying the action potentials with higher sweep speed.

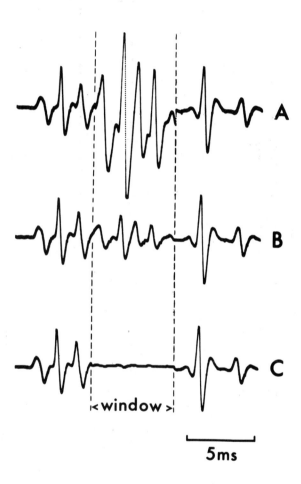

Fig. 10   Selective gain control in a part of a multi-spike recording by means of a "sweller".

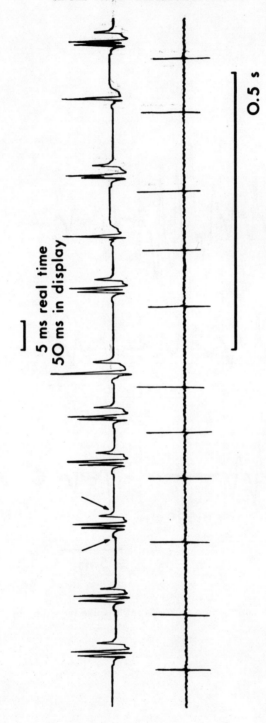

Fig. 11   Action potentials recorded by a pen recorder (lower trace), combined with a transient recorder which is read out at a slower time scale after each discharge (upper trace). Arrows indicate read-out time.

Sweller

It is sometimes of interest to either decrease or increase the amplitude of a portion of a multispike recording. A device can be used which allows a variable gain within a certain time window with optional location along the sweep and variable duration. The action potential can be attenuated to zero or increased by up to 10 times[20] (Fig. 10).

DOCUMENTATION

Some kind of *filming* procedure is usually the most convenient method of documentation. The "continuous" mode of film display is used to study firing pattern, and background activity, while the "raster" mode is convenient for studying, among other things, the shape of the action potentials with higher resolution. When a long-term recording is to be analysed and no equipment for running film is available a pen recorder can usually be used, but only to display the action potentials as events. Their shape is grossly distorted because of the inadequate frequency response of the pen recorder. With an *FM tape recorder* the time scale of the recording can be slowed down 10 to 100 times and now the frequency spectrum of the action potentials is suitable for a pen recording. Unfortunately the interdischarge intervals will also be increased by this factor, giving impracticably long paper recordings. With a *transient recorder* this time conversion can be done electronically and on-line. The short action potential of, say, 1 ms is written into a memory which is immediately read out at a slower rate, e.g. 50 times slower, which will give the potential a duration of 50 ms with its frequency spectrum reduced correspondingly. Now it can be recorded undistorted by means of an ink-jet recorder (Mingograph) or a pen recorder. Each action potential is slowed down by the chosen factor, but the interdischarge intervals will be unchanged, i.e. the recording on the paper will contain two different time scales. The "waiting" time between two discharges has been used for a slow display of the previous action potential (Fig. 11). Naturally action potentials stored by the *computer* can also be D/A converted and read out at a speed which is convenient for even slow plotters.

RECORDING PROCEDURES WITH DIFFERENT TYPES OF ACTIVATION

VOLUNTARY ACTIVITY

The electrode is inserted into weakly contracting muscle, usually in the middle third of its length. The motor point itself is avoided in order not to damage motor end-plates which might then give rise to abnormal recordings. The extreme ends of the muscles are not used lest unwanted factors come into play, such as tapering of muscle fibres with changed propagation velocity, abnormal motor unit topography with changed fibre density, and the possibility of larger temporal dispersion of individual muscle fibre action potentials in the same motor unit increasing the measured jitter at irregular innervation rates (page 56).

The recording surface should face the activated fibres as directly as possible, since 90 degrees of misrotation reduces the recording quality very significantly. The needle is slowly advanced into the muscle under the guidance of the loudspeaker. Technically, the best recordings are usually obtained from the superficial layers of the muscle, but none of the SFEMG parameters shows appreciable differences at different recording depths. The primary identification of the single fibre action potential is usually from its characteristic high-pitched crisp sound. Careful minimal corrections of the needle position including rotation are employed to make the potential amplitude as large as possible.

SFEMG is preferably performed with the muscle contracting minimally. Only one or few motor units within the uptake area of the electrode are then activated. If distant activity is recorded, the patient should be asked to relax a little without switching off the motor unit under study. Depending on the muscle, the recording position within the muscle and the skill of the patient, an undistorted recording is usually obtained when the firing frequency of the muscle fibre studied is between 8 and 15 discharges per second. Below 8 per second (5 for leg and back muscles) the firing rate is usually irregular. Above a firing rate of 15 discharges per second other recruited motor units usually interfere with the one under consideration. This range of firing rates introduces a bias towards lower threshold tonic motor units, which is also true for MUP studies with concentric needle electrodes.

The amplifier gain is usually set to 0.2 to 1 mV per division and the sweep speed initially to 0.5 to 1 ms per division. Some of the commonly used muscles and their relevant characteristics are now briefly discussed. The technique is in principle the same as that used in conventional electromyography; for SFEMG values see tables 4 and 5, pages 54 and 69.

Extensor digitorum communis (EDC) is used in many types of study. It is easy to activate, and age-dependent changes appear relatively later (after 70 years). It is conveniently examined with the prone forearm lying on the couch or the arm of a chair. The patient is asked to raise his middle finger slightly and the needle is inserted perpendicularly through the skin into the palpably contracting muscle. If repeated investigations are made in the same patient over weeks or months, different fingers may be raised on different occasions, in order to avoid recording from areas damaged by earlier needle penetrations. Multiple potentials are found in this muscle more easily than, for example, in *biceps brachii*, whereas single fibre action potentials are readily obtained in the latter. *Brachioradialis* has a well-defined end-plate zone which makes it particularly useful in studies in which nerve structures should be avoided, for example direct muscle stimulation. In this muscle the chance of recording fibre pairs with low jitter as well as pairs with long interspike intervals is higher than in many other muscles. *Frontalis* is best examined by inserting the needle horizontally from a lateral position, the patient then raising his eyebrows. The range of recruitment thresholds is fairly small in this muscle, so that many motor units are activated at once. It is relatively easy to obtain multiple potentials, and the mean interspike interval tends to be longer than in most other muscles (see page 70). *Quadriceps femoris* usually shows recruitment of motor units at low innervation rates. *Tibialis anterior* is apt to undergo secondary changes due to age and local compression of the supplying nerve, which must be taken into consideration. The ability to maintain regular motor unit firing rates as low as 4 discharges/second is not uncommon in this muscle.

ELECTRICAL STIMULATION

Nerve Trunk Stimulation

The motor unit can be activated by electrical stimulation of the motor axons with a *surface electrode* or a *needle electrode* near the nerve, or with a *micro-electrode* inside the nerve. With any of the three methods it is possible to stimulate only a few axons, but selective stimulation is most easily achieved with an intraneural electrode.

With the recording electrode in an appropriate muscle, single muscle fibre action potentials can be recorded. When many axons are activated a multispike response is obtained, showing a slight latency variation for each component individually. With decreasing stimulation strength the different components drop out, individually or several at a time. This is often preceded by a slight increase in latency and a significant increase in latency variation at consecutive stimuli[62] (Fig. 12). An intermediate stage of intermittent blocking with all-or-nothing behaviour of the spikes is seen. Finally, usually at a stage when little or no twitch is seen in the muscle, one or two components belonging to the same motor unit (appearing and disappearing simultaneously when the stimulus strength is changed in fine steps) are recorded.

In the normal muscle most of the latency variation occurring on suprathreshold stimulation of a particular axon is thought to arise at the neuromuscular junction (see jitter, page 33). The additional latency variability at threshold stimulus is due to variation in site and time of initiation of the impulse in the stimulated nerve fibre. When the rate of stimulation is below 10–20 Hz and the strength is suprathreshold, the mean latency and variability remain unchanged even during prolonged stimulation. At continuous high stimulation rates, e.g. 20–50 Hz — different for individual motor units — there is a progressive prolongation of the latency, accompanied by increasing latency variability and followed by intermittent blocking. This is probably due mainly to reduced excitability at the site of stimulation of the nerve fibre, and partly to subnormality of the remaining distal portion of the nerve

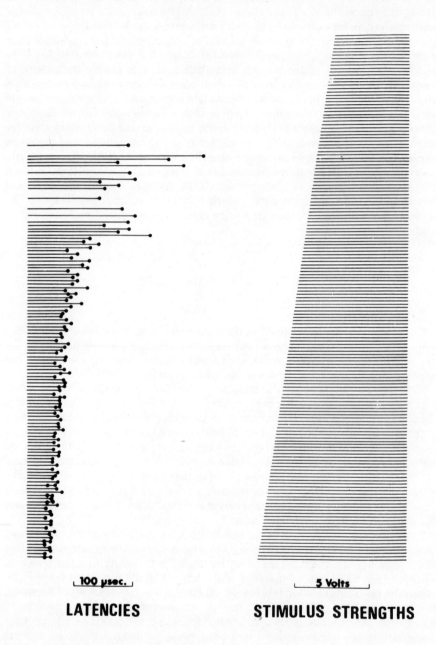

LATENCIES   **STIMULUS STRENGTHS**

Fig. 12   Recruitment of single fibre response at increasing stimulus strength on
nerve stimulation. Note the changes in latency and jitter (From Stålberg,
Trontelj and Trontelj, 1973).

fibre and the muscle fibre. The motor end-plate function is probably little affected at these stimulation rates. The subnormality at the site of stimulation may be temporarily overcome by increasing the stimulus amplitude or duration.

Intramuscular Nerve Stimulation

Using a stimulating needle electrode it is possible to activate the intramuscular axon branches. In general, the same phenomena can be seen as described above. The advantage with this type of stimulation is its selectivity: it is easier to activate single motor axons or axonal branches. Due to antidromic propagation of the nerve impulse and its invasion of other branches of the axon the whole motor unit is activated by the mechanism of axon reflexes[59] (see page 151).

When activated by axon reflexes the single muscle fibre action potentials of a motor unit are more dispersed in time and may appear in a different sequence from when they are activated at a more proximal site along the undivided motor axon, or by voluntary contraction.

Sometimes the latency variation is extremely small, indicating that the muscle fibre is activated directly (see below).

To obtain good recordings the positions of both the stimulating and recording electrodes have to be adjusted. A small, light-weight single fibre EMG electrode may retain its precise position for long periods if the connecting cable is fixed to the skin.

Direct Muscle Fibre Stimulation

If the stimulating electrode is positioned near the end of the muscle fibres, far enough from the nerve and the motor end-plate, or if the muscle is curarized or denervated, it is possible to activate muscle fibres directly by an electrical stimulus[77]. This is particularly the case with long stimulation pulses (1–100 ms) and particularly triangular pulses, where the difference in the rate of accommodation between nerve and muscle fibre favours the latter. Another way is to use bipolar stimulation, in which case muscle fibres can be stimulated directly even with short pulses (down to 0.05 ms). The evidence for direct muscle fibre stimulation in the normal muscle is the very small latency variation (less than 5 μs, MCD, see page 41) at suprathreshold stimulus strength. At decreasing stimulation strength the latency tends to increase more than on nerve stimulation (an order of 5–10 ms as compared with less than 2 ms for the nerve, when stimulating at low rates). The jitter increases more at threshold muscle stimulation than at threshold nerve stimulation (Fig. 13).

REFLEX ACTIVATION

In addition to voluntary activation and electrical stimulation of motor axons and muscle fibres, reflex activation can be used to study different SFEMG parameters. This includes well defined responses such as H-reflex, tendon jerk, blink reflex, flexion reflex, or just reflex facilitation procedures intended to support insufficient voluntary effort, such as muscle stretching, muscle vibration and cutaneous stimulation. These may be used in young children or when voluntary activity is difficult or impossible. The oscilloscope sweep is triggered as usual by the muscle fibre activity or, when convenient, by the given stimulus.

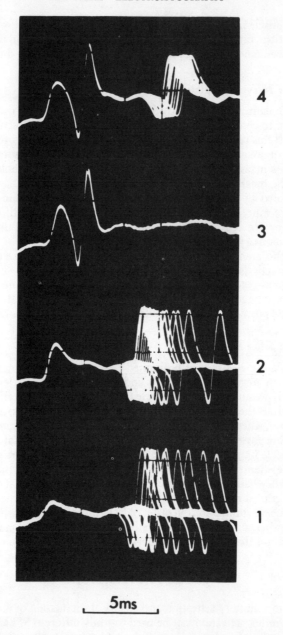

Fig. 13 Electrical stimulation of single muscle fibres. Lower trace, two fibres are activated, one supramaximally with low jitter and the other at its threshold, showing large jitter. In upper trace, the stimulus strength has been increased slightly, being now supramaximal for both fibres, but submaximal for a newly recruited fibre.

"MARKING" OF THE MOTOR UNIT

In some studies it is necessary to ensure that selective recordings from different sites in the muscle are made from the same motor unit. In other recordings it is necessary to distinguish the activity of one particular motor unit from interference by many others. This can be done by means of SFEMG and examples will be given of situations in which this method is used.

SINGLE FIBRE RECORDING

When single fibre action potentials from many muscle fibres belonging to the same motor unit are to be studied using different electrode positions, the problem arises of making certain that the recorded fibres really belong to the same motor unit. This can be done by monitoring the potentials from one fibre in the motor unit with a single fibre electrode, the activity of which is used to trigger the oscilloscope (trigger electrode, Fig. 14 A). With another SFEMG electrode (test electrode) a position is sought in which the recorded activity is time-locked to that from the trigger electrode during consecutive voluntary discharges. This indicates that the two electrodes are recording from muscle fibres belonging to the same motor unit. With the triggering electrode in constant position the test electrode can be used for recording from many different parts of the motor unit.

CONCENTRIC NEEDLE RECORDING

The test electrode can also be a concentric needle electrode. With a constant position of the triggering SFEMG electrode the electrical activity from one particular motor unit can be recorded from many positions in the muscle and the difference in shape of the so called motor unit potential can be demonstrated. The combined electrode described earlier, with small and large side port recording surfaces (the "macro-micro" electrode) may be used similarly, triggering on activity from the small selective electrode in order to study a larger population of fibres in the same motor unit with the large electrode surface. The use of a delay line is necessary to make possible the detection of action potentials preceding the triggering potential.

SURFACE ELECTRODE RECORDING

Voluntary motor unit activity can be recorded with surface electrodes, for example by recording between two silver strip electrodes (5 × 60 mm), one positioned across the belly of the muscle and the other over an indifferent area. The contribution to the surface EMG from a selected individual motor unit can be determined by feeding the surface-recorded signal via a delay line to an averager triggered by a reference single fibre action potential picked up by a SFEMG electrode (Fig. 14 B). In contrast to the technique described by McComas, Fawcett, Campbell and Sica (1971), this method is used for voluntarily activated muscle, which means that many different muscles can

31

be tested. Furthermore, each individual motor unit action potential is recorded separately and not superimposed on earlier recruited motor units. Considerably more than 10 motor units can be recorded in each tested muscle. The amplitudes range in EDC from 10 to 80 μV (mean 27 μV).

MOTOR UNIT TWITCH TENSION

In the same way the mechanical output from voluntarily activated muscle can be recorded and averaged, using single-fibre recording as the time reference. A similar technique has been described by Milner-Brown, Stein and Yemm (1973a), who used a concentric needle electrode as a reference.

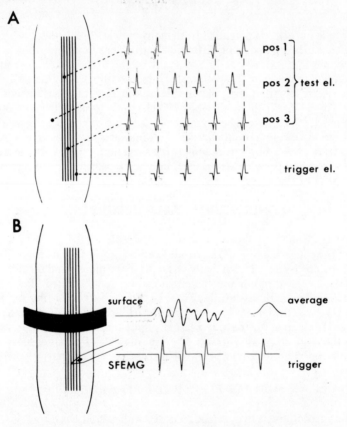

Fig. 14   A single fibre is recorded with a SFEMG electrode.
A. Another electrode can be positioned to find time-locked activity, i.e. fibres from the same motor unit, (pos. 1 and 3). In position 2 another motor unit is recorded.
B. Surface response can be averaged, time-related to the single fibre response to demonstrate the contribution to the surface response from the same motor unit.

SFEMG PHENOMENA AND PARAMETERS

JITTER AND IMPULSE BLOCKING

Electrical Stimulation

When a nerve fibre is stimulated repetitively well above the threshold and responses are recorded from a single muscle fibre there is a latency variability of the order of tens of μs. This is called the *jitter* and is due to variability in transmission time between the point at which the nerve is stimulated and the position along the muscle fibre at which the action potentials are recorded. (The term "Jitter" is adopted from the technical literature, where it denotes instability in an oscilloscope display due to a varying trigger level or an unstable time-base generator, c.f. German: Zitter). In the normal case, with suprathreshold stimuli, the variability in transmission time along the nerve fibre tested with microneurography (Torebjörk, personal communication) and along the muscle fibre tested at direct stimulation is less than 3 μs (MCD, see page 55). Thus the main source of the jitter in normal muscle on electrical stimulation of the nerve is considered to be the motor end-plate. This jitter may be due to small variations in the amplitude and thus steepness of the rising slope of the end-plate potential, causing it to reach the trigger level after a variable time interval, or it may be due to small fluctuations in the firing threshold, which would result in a variable neuromuscular transmission time even when the end-plate potential remains constant (Fig. 15).

The stimulation technique may be used when patients are unconscious or too young to co-operate, and in specific situations such as complete nerve conduction block or myasthenia gravis.

When using nerve trunk stimulation for studying jitter at the motor end-plate one should be aware that the local threshold for the electrical stimulus may gradually rise, particularly at higher stimulation rates, resulting in a progressive increase in jitter and in blocking due to subliminal stimulation. This can be proved by a moderate increase in stimulus strength, which returns the jitter to its initial values and does away with blocking (Fig. 16).

Moreover, when at threshold stimulation some responses fail to occur, this results in firing rate irregularity and a consequent further increase in jitter due to changing muscle fibre propagation velocity (see page 74); this is particularly conspicuous at higher stimulation rates (e.g. above 5 Hz). If the purpose of the study is to measure the motor end-plate jitter, the stimulus strength should be made suprathreshold for the axon to the recorded single fibre; the jitter does not decrease by further increasing the stimulus strength. It is important that no additional muscle fibres from adjacent motor units with a similar latency are activated at the same time since interfering action potentials could either increase or decrease the jitter of the summated action potential, depending on the stability of the disturbing single fibre action potentials. Normal values of the latency variability are of the order of 5–20 μs (MCD, see page 41).

When the nerve is stimulated intramuscularly the same phenomena in general are

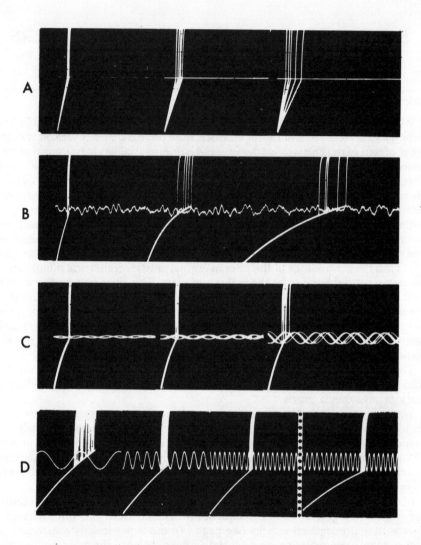

Fig. 15   The possible factors involved in the variability of the neuromuscular
transmission time. A: Variation in amplitude (and hence slope) of EPP's.
Three degrees of variability are shown. B: Fluctuation in the threshold for
depolarisation of muscle fibre membrane (trigger level) producing
different degrees of jitter at different EPP amplitude. C: Different
amplitude of trigger level variation results in different jitter for the same
EPP slope. D: Different frequencies of trigger level fluctuation. At high
frequency fluctuation the effect of lowering the EPP is small as shown in
the last example. Simulation experiment (From Stålberg, Schiller and
Schwartz, 1975).

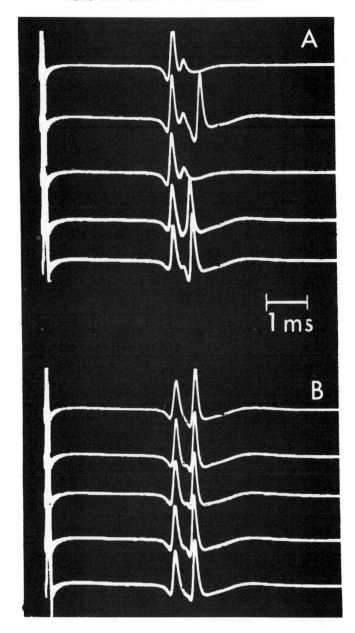

Fig. 16   The effect of submaximal axonal stimulation in normal subjects. In A there
is a variation in latency and blocking on two occasions of the second large
component. In B with increased stimulation strength there is a consistent
response with a similar latency (From Schwartz and Stålberg, 1975).

seen. One cause of erroneously high jitter should be mentioned: when measuring the jitter of a multiple potential of a single motor unit (indicated by simultaneous drop-out at decreasing stimulus), care must be taken to make the stimulus supramaximal for all components, since some may be activated not by axon reflexes but through activation of their own nerve twigs at a different distance from the stimulating electrode, hence with a different threshold stimulus strength. Sometimes the stimulus-response latency variation is very small, less than 5 μs. This is taken as an indication of direct muscle fibre stimulation.

Voluntary Activation

Jitter measurements can also be made in voluntarily activated muscle, in which case activity from two muscle fibres innervated by the same axon must be recorded and one action potential used as a reference (Fig. 17).

The mean interpotential interval (MIPI) is a value expressing the difference in conduction times along the two paths and thus reflects not only differing conduction velocities in nerve branches and muscle fibres, but also the difference in their anatomical lengths.

When the first action potential is made to trigger the oscilloscope sweep, the jitter is seen as a small variability in interpotential interval at consecutive discharges, i.e. the second action potential appears on the oscilloscope screen with a variable delay after the first action potential.

Thus, when motor units are voluntarily activated the jitter now results from variations in the *difference* in conduction times taken by impulses from the nerve branching point (b) via the motor end-plates along each muscle fibre to the recording site (E). Since one of the two responses is taken as the time reference, the combined variability is displayed by the other response and the recorded jitter can be expressed mathematically; $\sqrt{\text{jitter}_1^2 + \text{jitter}_2^2}$, as the two variabilities are independent and have approximately Gaussian distributions. (This is the jitter value used in *all* recordings at voluntary activation, and for example given in table 4 page 54).

In normal muscle and at a regular innervation frequency the jitter arises mainly at the motor end-plate. The magnitude of the jitter reflects the safety factor of the motor end-plate relative to curare, and after injection of a given dose of this drug those motor end-plates with the highest initial jitter show the greatest changes (see page 93). The jitter is thus correlated to a physiological property of the motor end-plate, probably the size of the end-plate potential relative to the firing threshold of the fibre.

Some part of the normal jitter may be caused by non-synaptic variability, notably in the muscle fibre.

The propagation velocity along a muscle fibre changes slightly in relation to the preceding impulse interval (velocity recovery function, VRF, page 74). For a short preceding interval the propagation velocity is higher than for an impulse following a long interval. A mutual difference of propagation velocity values of about 0.5–1% for consecutive discharges is seen in normal muscle (page 74).

When the conduction time along the two muscle fibres from the motor end-plate to the recording site is roughly the same, the interpotential interval is small. This is actually the case in most recordings, most of the interpotential interval values being

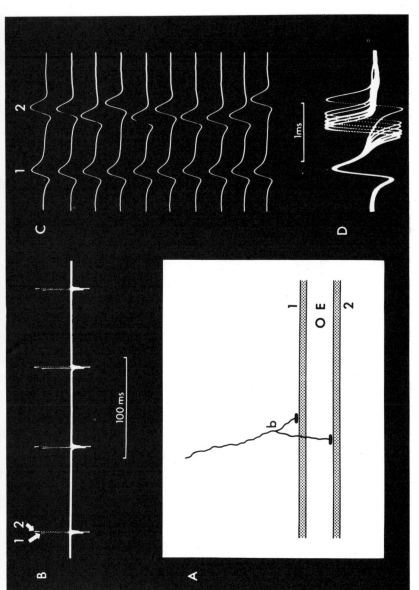

Fig. 17 A. Schematic explanation of the recording conditions for jitter measurement in voluntarily activated muscle. The single fibre EMG needle electrode is brought to a position from where it is possible to record from a pair of muscle fibres (I and II) innervated by the same motor axon. B shows the action potential pair firing at low degree of voluntary effort, C shows the two potentials at a higher sweep speed with the sweep triggered by the first potential and moving down after each discharge, and D shows several discharges superimposed to demonstrate changes in the interpotential intervals (the neuromuscular jitter).

SAME VELOCITY , DIFFERENT DISTANCES

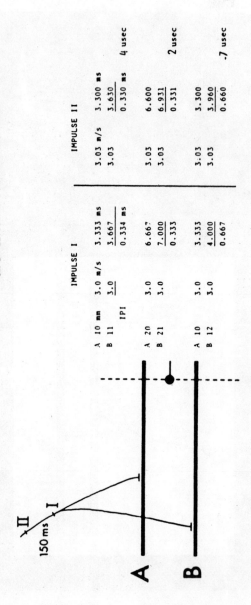

		IMPULSE I			IMPULSE II			
A 10 mm	3.0 m/s	3.333 ms			3.03 m/s	3.300 ms		
B 11	3.0	3.667			3.03	3.630		
IPI		0.334 ms				0.330 ms		4 usec
A 20	3.0	6.667			3.03	6.600		
B 21	3.0	7.000			3.03	6.931		
		0.333				0.331		2 usec
A 10	3.0	3.333			3.03	3.300		
B 12	3.0	4.000			3.03	3.960		
		0.667				0.660		.7 usec

PROPAGATION VELOCITY OF SECOND IMPULSE INCREASED BY 1%
CAUSING DECREASED INTERPOTENTIAL INTERVAL

Table 1. Effect of velocity recovery function on interpotential interval (IPI) for identical change in propagation velocity but different distances travelled by the impulse. The computed change in IPI for the second impulse for three theoretical sets of data is shown on the right.

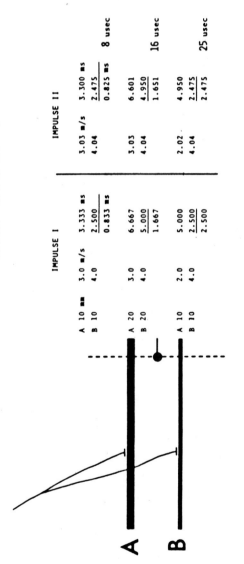

SAME DISTANCE , DIFFERENT VELOCITIES

	IMPULSE I			IMPULSE II		
A 10 mm	3.0 m/s	3.333 ms		3.03 m/s	3.300 ms	
B 10	4.0	2.500		4.04	2.475	
		0.833 ms			0.825 ms	8 usec
A 20	3.0	6.667		3.03	6.601	
B 20	4.0	5.000		4.04	4.950	
		1.667			1.651	16 usec
A 10	2.0	5.000		2.02	4.950	
B 10	4.0	2.500		4.04	2.475	
		2.500			2.475	25 usec

PROPAGATION VELOCITY OF THE SECOND IMPULSE INCREASED BY 1%
CAUSING DECREASED INTERPOTENTIAL INTERVAL.

Table 2. Effect of velocity recovery function on interpotential interval for different propagation velocities along the two fibres but identical distances travelled by the impulse.

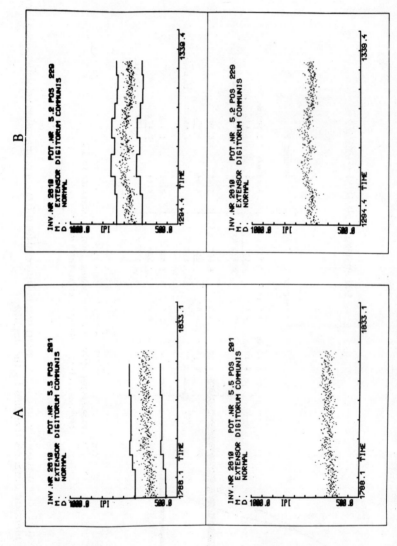

Fig. 18 Sequential histogram of interpotential intervals in two recordings (A and B) from a normal case. Slow trends are superimposed on the short term variability. The two lines indicate MIPI ± 4 MCD computed from each 50 discharges. (These limits are sometimes used to automatically reject wrong data, e.g. from interfering action potentials of other fibres).

less than 1 ms in the normal muscle. Since the two fibres belong to the same motor unit and are both affected by the same prior discharge the changes in the two conduction times due to this discharge will largely cancel each other out, provided that the propagation velocity changes are similar in the two fibres. In a hypothetical situation (tables 1 and 2) with reasonable assumptions about distance between motor end-plates (less than 2 mm), conduction velocity, strength of VRF and irregularity of innervation rate, the variability in the interpotential interval which is added to the neuromuscular jitter is usually less than 10 μs. If the mean interpotential interval is long (of the order of many milliseconds) and is due to widely separated motor end-plates or to pronounced differences in muscle fibre conduction velocities, the short term changes along the muscle fibre will not cancel out. The variability at moderately irregular innervation rates can be as much as 50 μs, which is added to the neuromuscular jitter.

In pathological cases with widely separated motor end-plates, great differences in propagation velocity and pronounced VRF (page 74), variations in propagation velocity along the muscle fibres may produce changes in consecutive interpotential intervals by more than 100 μs.

The effect on the jitter of variable muscle fibre propagation velocity is naturally not seen when using electrical stimulation at a constant frequency. At irregular stimulation frequency and on voluntary activation, the contribution of this interval-dependent variability to the measured jitter can be determined mathematically (see MSD below).

Calculation of the Jitter

The time variability for consecutive discharges can be mathematically expressed as the *standard deviation (SD)* around a mean value (MIPI), but there are sometimes slow trends superimposed on the short-term random variation (Fig. 18); these are mainly due to different degrees of slowing of the propagation velocity along the two muscle fibres during continuous activity or to minor changes in action potential shape resulting from slight displacement of the recording electrode. Such trends would increase the calculated SD, which would then not be an accurate measure of the jitter. Another way of expressing the variability is to calculate the consecutive interpotential interval differences and to use the *Mean value of Consecutive Differences (MCD)*,[10] expressed in absolute values, over a number of discharges (usually 20–50). In Gaussianly distributed material without trends, MCD equals 1.13 SD. The MCD value will measure only the short term variability and is practically unaffected by slow trends, which makes it more suitable for jitter evaluation than SD. Other measures can also be used, such as SD around a sliding mean value. MCD was chosen because it was simple to handle when building analogue or digital jittermeters, and it measures the jitter accurately.

In certain pathological situations the interpotential interval is influenced by the preceding interdischarge interval (Fig. 19). In this case the calculated MCD would include additional variability besides the neuromuscular jitter, i.e. that due to the velocity recovery function (page 74). In order to eliminate this factor, the measured interpotential intervals are sorted according to the preceding interdischarge intervals in increasing order, after which the mean value of consecutive differences in this new sequence is calculated. This parameter is termed *MSD*, i.e. *Mean*

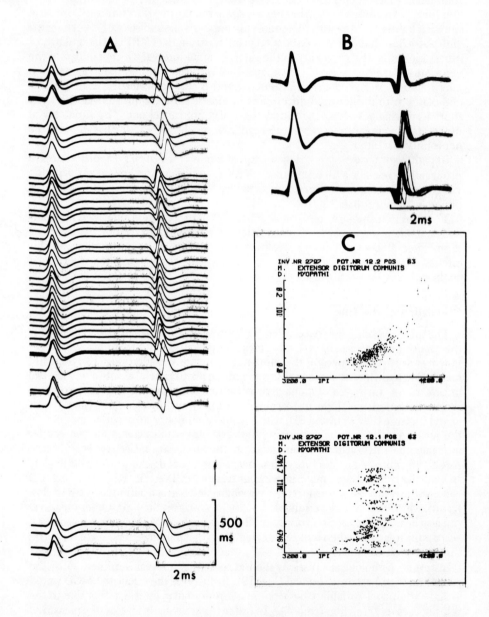

Fig. 19 A muscle fibre pair from a patient with muscular dystrophy showing dependence of interpotential interval on the preceding interdischarge interval. A and B, actual recording; C, computer analysis.

Sorted-data Difference. In practical work, the quotient MCD/MSD is calculated as an index: when this value exceeds 1.25, the variability is influenced by interdischarge intervals to the extent that MSD should be used instead of MCD for evaluation of the neuromuscular jitter. If the value of the index is lower than 0.80, this indicates that slow trends are present. In this case the MCD value should be used. In the range 0.80–1.25 the MCD value is used.

Practical Ways of Measuring the Jitter

Usually the interval measurement is made from the baseline intersection point on the triggering action potential to the corresponding point on preceding or successive spike components. Background activity, movements of the needle and physical noise should be kept as low as possible since they may considerably increase the estimated jitter (page 51). When the two action potentials interfere with each other (the second potential riding on the first), the jitter measured as described will be either overestimated or underestimated (see page 51). In this case time measurements can be made between the peaks. Different techniques for measuring the jitter have been developed:

1. Computer analysis — The consecutive intervals between the two action potentials can be measured and the jitter can be calculated conveniently and accurately with a time interval counter or with the real-time clock in a computer.

With time interval counter: When a time interval counter with digital output is available the following procedure can be used (Fig. 20). The potential pair is fed to a dual-beam dual-time base oscilloscope, which is triggered by the first component, and to the counter. The counter can be activated only during the time of the oscilloscope gate A, thus preventing spurious potentials from being counted. The multiple action potential is displayed on sweep A and the selected jittering spike on the delayed sweep B. The counter is stopped only by signals appearing during the time of gate B. In this case any component of a multiple spike potential can be selected to stop the counter. The start and the stop trigger levels should be set as close to the zero intersection point on the fast rising slope of the action potential as possible. If an action potential does not appear during sweep B an impulse blocking is registered. The start and stop points are indicated on the oscilloscope as intensified spots produced by pulses from the counter connected to the Z-axis of the oscilloscope. When no dual-beam oscilloscope is available two "time windows" can be electronically generated with variable position (determined by the horizontal voltage of the potential triggered oscilloscope) and duration. In the same way as above, counter start is only possible during the first time window and stop only during the second.

Each discharge is analysed and its value in binary form is serially fed to the computer via an interface. In addition to the time interval it is convenient to have a time clock. This is read simultaneously with the interval value to provide information about discharge rate.

Without time interval counter: It is also possible to use an analogue input (action potential) to the computer and its internal real-time clock for interval measurements. The clock can be started by oscilloscope gate A (synchronous with the triggering action potential) and stopped by a second action potential appearing during the time of gate B.[31] Instead of feeding the action potentials themselves to the computer

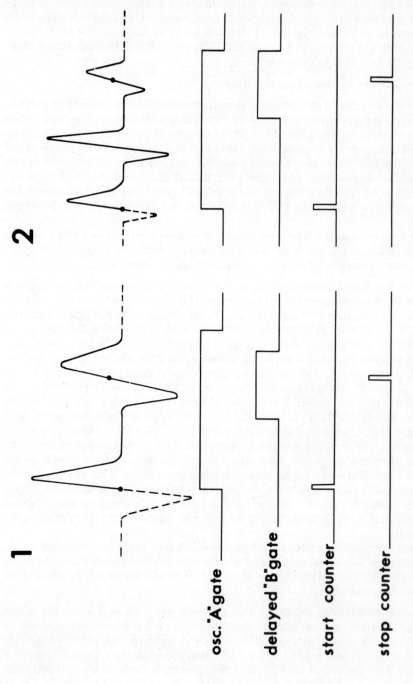

Fig. 20 Time interval measurements by means of a counter. Start at oscilloscope gate A triggered by the first action potential. Stop on any chosen action potential appearing during the time of gate B the position of which can be optically chosen.

input, the action potentials can be transformed into square pulses (e.g. the gate pulses at fast sweep of the oscilloscope) and these pulses are then used to start and stop the real-time clock. In this way the triggering manoeuvre is accomplished at the recording equipment instead of at the input to the computer.

Display: The jitter is analysed as the MCD and MSD values. As mentioned above, time windows are set as limits for acceptable data. If no limits are used some potential pairs will be recorded with erroneously high jitter due to false triggering. The jitter values can be displayed as sequential histograms. In this way, the limits used can easily be checked and trends can be detected. Nonsequential histograms may also be displayed, giving a general impression of the size of the jitter; bimodal jitter distributions can thus be detected more easily. The jitter values can also be continuously displayed during an investigation. With the data stored, an interdischarge interval vs interpotential interval plot can be made to test the jitter dependence on the preceding interval. Interdischarge intervals can be plotted for the study of the innervation rate. In addition, the interdischarge interval plot can be used to detect occasional neuromuscular blocking when recording is made from a single spike; in this case, some intervals are multiples of the shorter intervals (Fig. 21).

Jittermeter: A special jittermeter has been built with a microprocessor as the computing unit, allowing one to obtain all the major SFEMG parameters[65]. Time measurements are made with an internal clock and the results are displayed on LED-displays, oscilloscope, X-Y plotter and a printer-plotter.

2. Nonsequential histograms of interpotential intervals. The action potentials can be transformed into short square pulses (2–5 μs) and then fed into equipment for interval histogramming (Fig. 22, 3). This gives a histogram of the time intervals. As long as no trends are present (detected by checking during the continuous recording) a value of SD can be given[66,68] or a conversion to MCD made to express the jitter (Blom and Ringqvist, 1970).The two square pulses representing the action potential can also be fed into a signal averager with the first potential used as a trigger impulse. The varying position of the second will produce a histogram of the intervals. In both instances a time resolution (address time) of ten μs or less is necessary.

3. Sequential histogram of interpotential intervals. The action potentials can be transformed into square pulses and fed to the z-axis of the oscilloscope (intensity modulation). The oscilloscope sweep is triggered by the first impulse. When the horizontal sweep is moved downwards the second action potential will be seen on the oscilloscope as a dot with variable x-position corresponding to the interpotential interval (Fig. 22, 2). In the same way as with superimposition, a range of values for any number of consecutive discharges can be measured.

4. Photographic superimposition. By superimposing on film a small number (2–10) of consecutive discharges and measuring the range of interpotential intervals with a sweep speed normally not slower than 200 μs/div., a measure of the variability can be obtained (Fig. 22, 1). The range should be measured between identical points on the fast positive-negative deflections of the action potentials. Recordings with unstable triggering should be discarded. The range value can be subsequently transformed into values numerically comparable to MCD values in order to obtain a comparable measure for the jitter between different laboratories. A suitable way is to

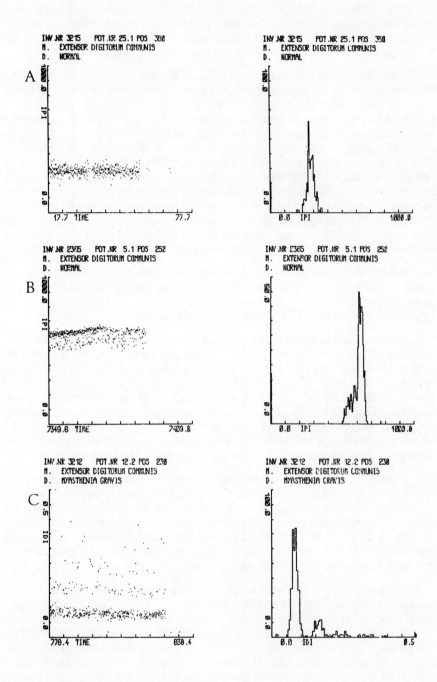

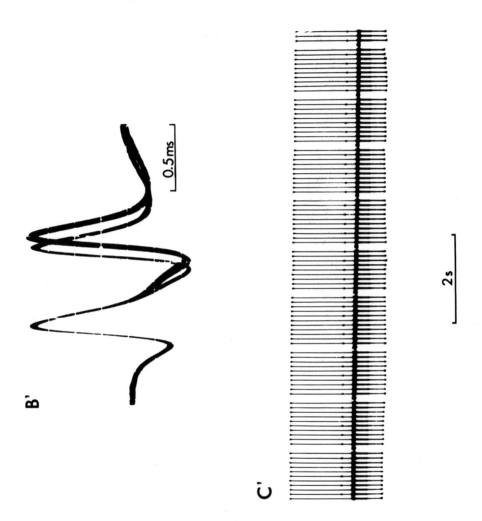

Fig. 21 (see facing page) Sequential and nonsequential histograms of *interpotential* intervals in a case of normal jitter (A) and in a case of a bimodal-distributed jitter (B), also seen in the actual recording above. C shows histograms of *interdischarge* intervals in a case of an intermittently blocking single fibre action potential. B[1] and C[1] are samples of actual recording.

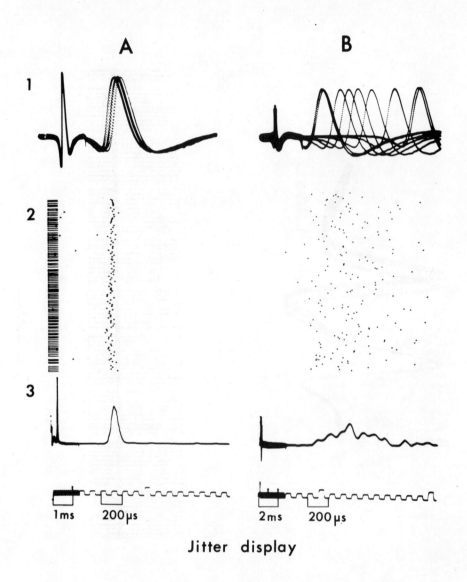

Jitter display

Fig. 22   Jitter display in a normal (A) and an abnormal (B) potential pair. 1. Actual recordings with dual sweep time and superimposition. Sequential and nonsequential histograms obtained by feeding short square pulses (5 μs) coinciding with the zero intersection point of the action potentials to the Z-axis, i.e. intensity modulation of an oscilloscope (2) and into an averager (3).

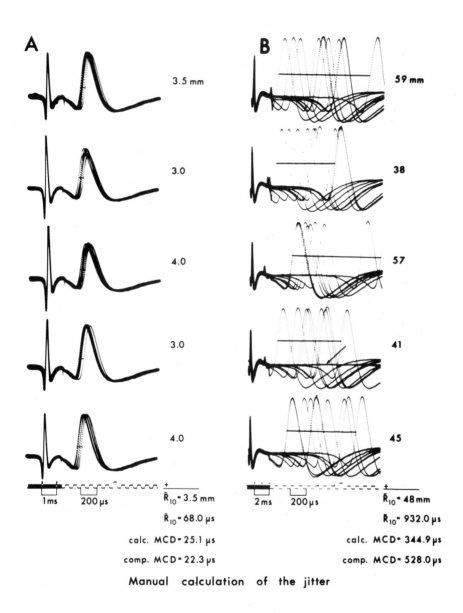

Manual calculation of the jitter

Fig. 23   Manual calculation of the jitter in a normal (A) and abnormal (B) action
potential pair. Five groups of 10 superimpositions are made and ranges of
interpotential interval variation are measured for each group. Mean value
is then calculated and multiplied by 0.37 to obtain an approximation to
MCD.

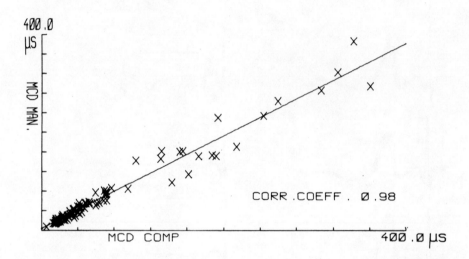

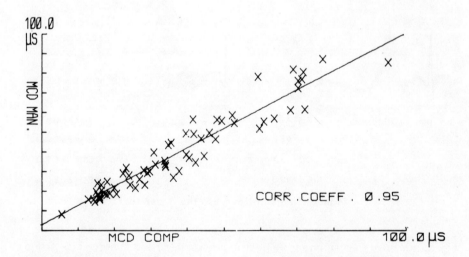

Fig. 24   Correlation between manual and computer calculation of the jitter. Lower part shows a smaller section of the upper part.

superimpose 10 discharges 5 times and calculate the mean range of 10 (mean R_{10}). MCD is then calculated according to the formula:

$MCD = R_{10} \times 0.37$ (table 3, Fig. 23)[10]. MCD estimated as described, from manual measurements of the superimposed potentials, is a good approximation to the MCD measured and calculated by computer (Fig. 24).

Jitter measure

	MCD	SD	R_2	R_3	R_4	R_5	R_6	R_7	R_8	R_9	R_{10}
Factor	1.00	1.13	1.00	0.67	0.55	0.49	0.45	0.42	0.40	0.38	0.37

Table 3. Conversion factors for obtaining MCD value from SD and mean ranges of variation of interpotential intervals in 2–10 consecutive discharges.

Error Sources in Jitter Measurement

The most accurate point for measuring jitter, propagation velocity and duration of multispike potentials is the zero intersection point of the action potential. This signifies the moment at which the recording surface is perpendicular to the passing depolarisation front. If the electrode is moved in relation to the fibre, the amplitude of the action potential decreases and the action potential tilts around this point (Fig. 25). This part of the action potential is therefore the least sensitive to movement artefacts, and the farther away from the baseline the measurement is made, the more movement artefact will change the amplitude and increase the jitter.

In both manual and automatic measurements the time reference point is usually described with an amplitude criterion. If the baseline is unstable (hum, noise, background muscle activity) the action potential is moving up and down and the measurements are made from varying parts of the action potential (Fig. 26). This is, naturally, especially true if a slow phase of the action potential be chosen, but it may also play a role when measurements are correctly made on the steep rising phase. If a 10 mV action potential with a 10–90% peak rise time of 100 μs is fluctuating by as much as 1 mV the reference point has moved 10 μs. A similar situation is inevitably faced when the two action potentials in a potential pair are interfering with each other and the second is "riding" on the first. A level-determined reference point gives an overestimation of the jitter. When the action potentials are separated by more than 100 μs, a prerequisite to any measurements, the first action potential will be moved positively, i.e. the measuring level will be reached later. The second potential will be moved negatively, i.e. its measuring level will be reached earlier and the interpotential value will be falsely shortened. At the next discharge their mutual interference is changed and the error mentioned above will have another magnitude. Thus, when the potentials are riding on each other the chosen time measuring points will move for each discharge, increasing the measured jitter. In this situation the peak of the action potential is the preferred reference point. This is particularly the case in recordings of complex action potentials with pronounced interference between the spike components (see computer analysis). When using the peak as reference this must be defined with the highest possible accuracy, preferably electronically (first derivative = 0).

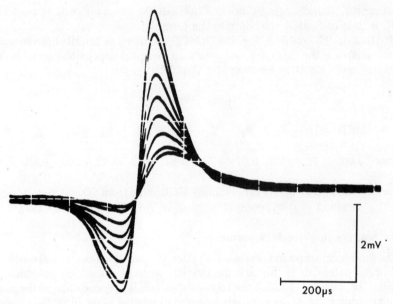

Fig. 25 "Tilting" of the action potential due to movement of the electrode as much as 280 μm (as determined by the multi-electrode).

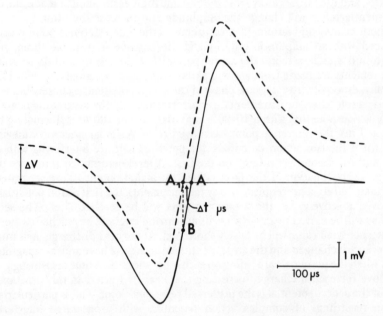

Fig. 26 Change in the trigger point set at a voltage level on an action potential from A to $A_1 = \Delta t$ μs at vertical displacement by ΔV. The new trigger point A_1 corresponds to point B on the action potential in the original position.

Normal Jitter Values on Voluntary Activity

In the normal muscle there is a considerable range of jitter values, and this also applies to motor end-plates belonging to a single motor unit. The jitter values are the same whether the recording is made close to the end-plate or close to the tendon. There is no correlation between the mean interpotential interval (MIPI) and the size of the jitter for MIPI values less than 4 ms, and this limit is only exceptionally exceeded in normal muscle.

The physiological degree of irregularity which occurs at steady contraction does not influence the jitter, but at very irregular innervation rates the jitter sometimes increases slightly (Tables 1 and 2). A decrease of the intramuscular temperature below 35°C increases the jitter in normal muscle by 1–3 μs/°C. At 25°C the jitter is about 80–100 μs. Increase in temperature between 35 and 38°C does not seem to decrease or increase the normal jitter value. The normal values range between 5 and 35–60 μs (MCD) for different muscles, with some exceptional values above this limit, not more than one in any subject tested (Fig. 27). For the same muscle there are also inter-individual differences (Fig. 28), possibly reflecting different safety factors in different individuals. No age-dependent changes were found in EDC muscle below the age of 70, when fibre density values (page 69) were normal. It is our impression that higher jitter values are found in the tibialis anterior after the age of 50, when they are usually associated with an increase in fibre density, and therefore probably indicate neurogenic changes. Concentric needle EMG of this muscle also shows increase in MUP amplitude after this age (Hayward, 1977). The extensor digitorum brevis muscle may show increased jitter and fibre-density values much earlier, even before the age of 20. The mean jitter value in a muscle of a single normal subject may differ from normal mean values for the population by as much as 30%. The mean jitter value in two normal subjects may differ significantly, by as much as 1 : 2. The range of jitter values in one individual is usually smaller than the range of the whole material in one muscle. Mean values and suggested upper normal limits in some muscles are given in Table 4. The upper limit has been defined as the highest value in the complete normal material after extreme individual values (exceeding mean + 5 SD) have been discarded. In none of the normal subjects was such an extreme value seen in more than one out of 20 recorded pairs. This implies that a jitter investigation of 20 potential pairs is considered normal if no more than one exceeds the given upper limits (even if this one shows blocking). Above the age of 70, more recordings may show high jitter. In some instances the mean jitter value repays attention even when all individual values are within normal limits. This can be the case in mild myasthenic involvements (Sanders, Howard and Johns, 1978) and also when the effect of drugs or environmental toxins is being studied or when the course of electrolyte disturbances is being followed in a given subject.

Long-Term Recording

It is sometimes possible to make continuous jitter recordings from one and the same potential pair for up to three hours at innervation rates between 10 and 15 per second. In the normal muscle there is no significant change in the jitter during recordings of this length.

In recordings at innervation rates over 30 per second the jitter does not show any

Muscles	Number of potential pairs	MCD — pooled data mean, SD	SD of MCD values from individual subjects mean, SD	Upper normal limit close to mean + 3SD
frontalis	258	20.4, 8.8	6.2, 2.3	45
(range of means for individual subjects)		(15.7 – 29.2)	(5.5 – 8.7)	
biceps	125	15.6, 5.9		35
EDC	759	24.6, 10.6	8.3, 3.2	55
(range of means for individual subjects)		(16.5 – 32.0)	(2.3 – 12.4)	
rectus femoris	73	31.0, 12.6		(65)* 60
tibialis anterior	153	32.1, 15.0		(75)* 60
EDB	29	85.3, 68.6		none

Table 4. Jitter (MCD) at voluntary activation in different muscles of normal subjects aged 10–70 years. The suggested upper limit has been chosen to Mean + 3 SD.

*Due to some extreme high values the data are not Gaussian distributed. A more appropriate upper normal limit is 60 μs.

In no one normal subject was there more than one value exceeding this limit.

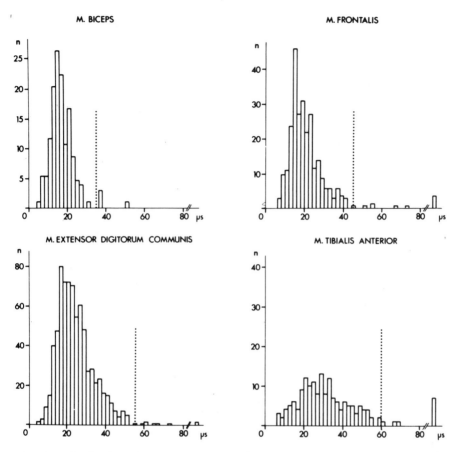

Fig. 27 Distribution of MCD values in different muscles in normal subjects. All individual data are included. The dotted line indicates the upper normal limit about which not more than one in 20 values was found in any one subject.

appreciable change during periods of up to 10 minutes, the longest tested before a subject has become fatigued.

Low Jitter

Sometimes very small jitter is obtained on voluntary contraction (less than 3–5 μs). This is considered to be due to recording from two branches of the same muscle fibre after muscle fibre splitting or fibre budding. In this situation no motor end-plate transmission is involved between the triggering and the second action potential. This is only exceptionally seen in the normal muscle but more often in muscular dystrophies. It is not yet clear whether actual splitting of a dystrophic muscle fibre always gives rise to low jitter, or whether a variability may arise along the abnormal muscle fibre.

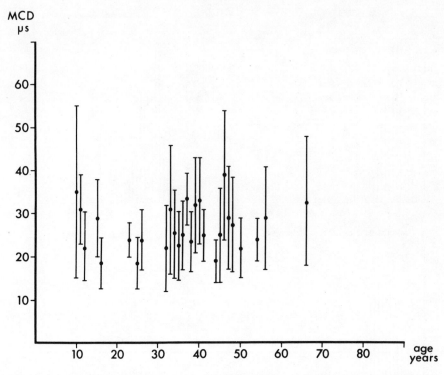

Fig. 28   A plot of MCD values (mean ± 1SD) in EDC muscle of some normal subjects
in different ages. There is no age-dependent change up to the age of 70
years, but there is considerable interindividual variation.

Jitter in Potential Pairs with Long Interpotential Intervals

The jitter is typically of Gaussian distribution and independent of innervation rate
and needle position in the muscle. When, however, the interpotential interval is more
than about 4 ms the length of the preceding interdischarge interval becomes
important. This is because conduction time at consecutive discharges changes with
varying interdischarge intervals, mainly along the muscle fibres (see VRF, page 74),
and to a lesser extent along the nerve fibre. The effect of short-term variability of
propagation velocity becomes so large as significantly to increase the measured jitter
at uneven innervation rates. This can be seen as a positive correlation between
interdischarge interval and the following inter-potential interval in one potential pair
at consecutive discharges (Fig. 19). Normal values given in table 4 are therefore valid
for interpotential intervals of less than 4 ms, which is in any case only exceptionally
exceeded in the normal recording. In this situation the MSD value (page 41) should
be calculated and for an MCD/MSD index over 1.25 the MSD value should be used.
At a uniform firing rate, such as in electrical stimulation of the motor axons, this
mechanism naturally does not operate. (Table 1 and Table 2)

Bimodal Jitter

In some recordings a double distribution of the interpotential intervals is seen[63], particularly when the mean interpotential interval is less than 1 ms (Fig. 29 A and B). This grouping around two mean values is less distinct when the distance between the peaks is small or when there are only few values in one of the two peaks. Bimodal jitter is seen in about one in 20 recordings from normal muscle. When it is recognised, by its typical sound or by the oscilloscope picture, the jitter should be measured at only one of the two positions or the recording discarded. An "abnormal" jitter in a normal muscle may be due to this type of phenomenon.

The mechanism responsible for the short-interval bimodal jitter could be subdepolarization of the second fibre by the electrical field of the immediately preceding action potential (deriving from the adjacent first fibre in the pair) causing a changed propagation velocity for some discharges. Another possibility is that the first fibre's action potential actually summates with the end-plate potential of the second, increasing it when it arrives at the correct moment. This is only possible when there is a critical time relationship between the action potentials of the two fibres, and therefore only occurs at short interpotential intervals, i.e. when action potentials in two adjacent muscle fibres are propagating almost simultaneously.

A similar phenomenon can be seen in reinnervation, where the jumps are longer (up to 16 ms has been seen). This may be due to uncertain impulse conduction in the poorly myelinated nerve twig during the process of remyelination. There may be a transitional stage between continuous conduction in the poorly myelinated nerve sprout and saltatory conduction in the mature nerve twig. Other explanations are possible. A long jump may be misinterpreted as an impulse blocking if the action potential is not observed in its new position in the complex potential under study (Fig. 29 C and D).

Increased Jitter and Blocking

Increased jitter may be due to abnormally low or abnormally variable end-plate potentials, and perhaps to variation in the depolarisation threshold of muscle-fibre membrane or to both (Fig. 15). In normal muscle an increased jitter can be seen at low temperatures, with ischaemia and during slight curarisation. With very few exceptions, the jitter is already increased by the time blocking of transmission occurs, i.e. before the muscle becomes weak. Typically, blocking starts when jitter values exceed 80–100 μs. If both motor end-plates are equally abnormal, the jitter value is higher when the first blocking occurs than when only one motor end-plate is involved.

Increased jitter in disease is usually due to disturbed neuromuscular junctions, as in myasthenia gravis[18], the myasthenic syndrome and electrolyte disturbances, but may also be due to disturbed conduction of nerve and muscle fibre impulses in certain pathological conditions[46]. This is of particular importance in cases of reinnervation and in muscular dystrophies. The jitter may be increased to several times the upper normal limit in recordings with impulse blocking, and may exceptionally reach 1000 μs, MCD (see under myasthenia gravis and myasthenic syndrome, pages 120–131). The range between the shortest and the longest interpotential interval in a series of consecutive discharges can be up to 4000 μs.

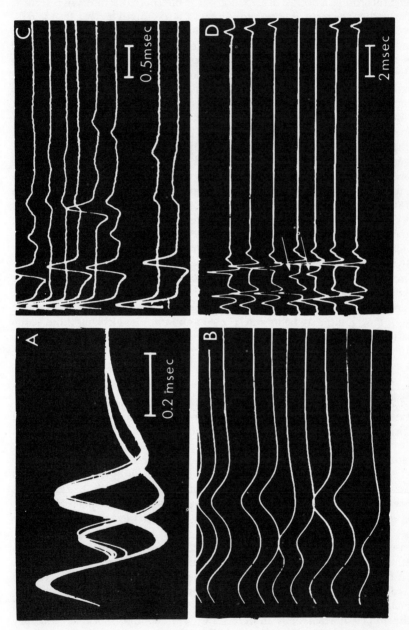

Fig. 29 Bimodal jitter. The interpotential interval alternates between two different mean values. A and B, example of a short-interval between the two positions, as seen in normal muscles. C and D, with long intervals between the two positions, obtained in cases with reinnervation. (From Thiele and Stålberg, 1974)

Concomitant Blocking

When a recording is made from three or more muscle fibres during voluntary activation, especially when there is peripheral reinnervation, two or more components may show intermittent simultaneous blocking in contrast to the previously described independent blocking of individual spikes. These potentials also show a large common jitter in relation to the other parts of the action potential-complex (Fig. 30). This phenomenon can be interpreted in at least two ways. If the jitter between the components which are intermittently disappearing together is abnormally small (less than 5 μs) the fault may lie at a single motor end-plate, which would mean that the spikes are generated by the branches of a split muscle fibre. A small interspike jitter is thus essential before this explanation can be entertained (see page 55). If on the other hand there is a jitter of more than 5 μs between the blocking components, another explanation is more likely: the phenomenon may then be due to an intermittent block in the common axonal branch supplying the muscle fibres from which the blocking action potentials are recorded. The common jitter in relation to the non-blocking spikes in the complex is due to the same mechanism, i.e. the unreliable axonal impulse conduction[55]. Axonal blocking can only be identified when at least three components are recorded. When the presence of axonal blocking is suspected it is important to check the triggering potential. If components 2 and 3 in a triple potential block, the first component remains the triggering potential. If components 1 and 2 block, the last component should be identified as the triggering one. If none of the original components is found to trigger the sweep at the moment of suspected "blocking", this is not axonal blocking but spurious triggering from another motor unit. When activity from two muscle fibres is recorded it is not possible to differentiate between neuromuscular and axonal jitter and blocking.

Just as in the neuromuscular blocking encountered in myasthenia gravis (see page 120), axonal blocking may increase during continuous activity and with increasing innervation rate, and may also give rise to some decrement in the surface-recorded responses to repetitive stimulation. It may also show a response to Tensilon[55], from which it follows that the presence of a decrement and of a positive Tensilon effect is not absolute proof of a synaptic transmission defect.

Phenomena Simulating Single-spike and Concomitant Blocking

False double potentials. Now and then the triggering potential is followed by a positive going, mainly monophasic potential with a longer rise-time and longer total duration than the normal single fibre action potential (Fig. 31). This potential often shows a large jitter and blocking and its delay from the triggering potential increases with increasing innervation rate. The reverse is also seen; with decreasing innervation rate it may approach the leading potential and sometimes join it so as to constitute a part of the main potential (making it triphasic) but now without jitter. With slight movements of the electrode it is sometimes possible to "shake off" this potential altogether. Occasionally two or three such potentials are seen to leave the main potential in succession.

This second triangular potential is believed to be generated by the same fibre as the triggering one, most likely by a mechanically damaged portion of the muscle fibre

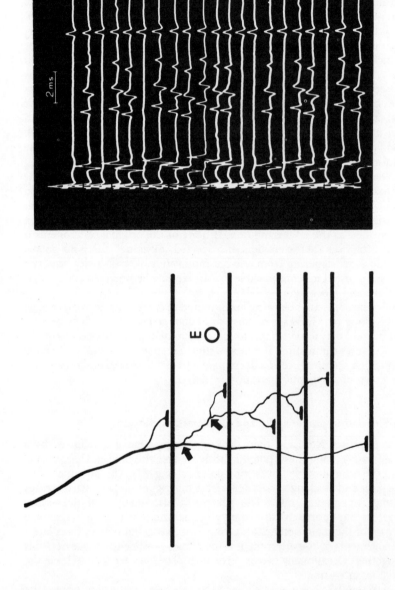

Fig. 30   Concomitant blocking. A recording from 6 muscle fibres from the same motor unit. The middle four spike components intermittently block together. They also show a large common jitter in relation to the remaining two components. The block is considered to be situated in the nerve twig common for the four blocking muscle fibres, that is, between the two arrows in the schematic drawing. (From Stålberg, Trontelj and Janko, 1974)

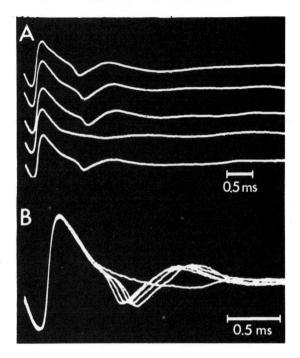

Fig. 31 "False double potential" probably due to damaged muscle fibre. The second broad monophasic deflection is not derived from a second muscle fibre and the recording is not accepted for jitter measurements.

membrane. This recording should not be used for jitter measurements. For fibre density measurements the false double potential should be counted as one single fibre action potential. It should be noted that when using a high pass filter of more than 500 Hz this monophasic potential may become bi- or tri-phasic. With random insertions such potentials can be obtained in up to 25% of recordings, or even more often when there is a hook at the electrode tip.

Extra-discharges (see also page 80). In some normal recordings of single or multiple action potentials, but particularly in pathological cases, some of the discharges are followed by an extra-discharge after 4–15 ms (Fig. 32). Some components may be missing in the second discharge due to refractoriness, and there may be changes in the shape of the individual spikes and in the interpotential intervals. The extra-discharge may thus differ in form from the original single or multiple potential and be misinterpreted as neuromuscular or axonal blocking. The amplitude of the individual spike components in the extra-discharge progressively falls to as low as 75% of the original at an interval of 4 ms (page 80). In some situations, especially in motor neurone disorders, an extra-discharge may follow every discharge over long periods, particularly when the innervation rate is below a certain critical level[54].

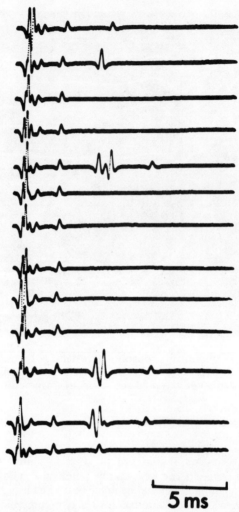

5 ms

Fig. 32 A multiple potential recording from a case of polymyositis. In three traces extradischarges are seen simulating concomitant blocking. The shape of the extradischarge is slightly changed due to the nerve and/or muscle fibres. In the first two and in the last trace only one component is repeated in the extradischarge.

"*Recruitment*". This is a rare phenomenon seen in the normal muscle. A new action potential may be recruited to fire in conjunction with previously discharging single or multiple action potential when the innervation rate exceeds certain value. The amplitude is low at first and the rise time prolonged; after a few discharges the amplitude increases, while the rise time and the interval to the original potential decrease. The jitter and potential shape may then be normal, except for inverted polarity in some cases. The significance of this finding is not quite clear, but it may be an artefact of the technique.

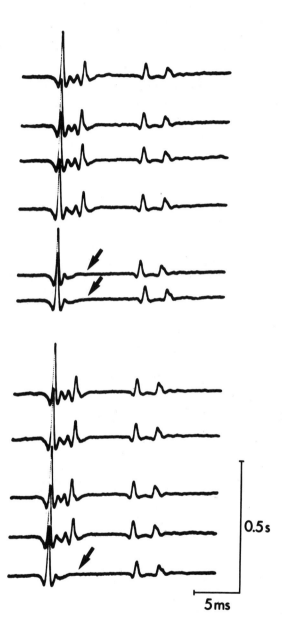

Fig. 33 Recruitment of additional action potentials to a multiple potential at increasing innervation rate in a case of Duchenne dystrophy.

In some cases of muscular dystrophy and polymyositis a similar phenomenon may be seen resembling axonal blocking. This is the synchronous recruitment of two or more additional spikes to a multiple action potential with increasing innervation rate[44] (Fig. 33). When the innervation rate is lowered the extra spikes disappear, thus reacting to changes in innervation rate in the opposite way to axonal blocking. This phenomenon is further discussed on page 146. It may indicate that impaired transmission in the axon or in a split fibre (when there is more than one component) is being overcome by the facilitation afforded by an increased firing rate. It could also be due to driving of the adjacent hyperexcitable muscle fibres by ephaptic transmission or central synchronization of different motor units, though the latter explanation is rather unlikely.

FIBRE DENSITY

By counting the number of single muscle fibres from one motor unit within the uptake area of the electrode in each of many electrode positions a measure of the mean fibre density within a motor unit can be calculated[57]. The electrical field of a muscle fibre can be recorded as an action potential with an amplitude more than 200 μV and a rise time less than 300 μs, at a distance of up to 150–300 μm, depending on fibre diameter (large fibres can be recorded from farther away than small fibres). In the normal adult muscle the average uptake radius is about 250–300 μm (Fig. 34, 35) when the above criteria are used. For bipolar recordings the uptake area is different and the technique and values given below apply to monopolar derivation.

Recording Technique

The electrode is randomly inserted in the muscle and the action potential from one fibre is made maximal by correction of the electrode position. One then counts the number of synchronous spike components which have an amplitude exceeding 200 μV and a rise time shorter than 300 μs when using a low frequency limit of 500 Hz at the amplifier. In order to detect a small action potential still fulfilling the above criteria and preceding a larger spike component, the trigger level of the oscilloscope must be set as low as 200 μV. It is more convenient to use a delay line of at least 5 ms and arrange stable triggering on a larger spike component, not necessarily the first in the recorded response. The sweep speed should be slow enough to cover at least 5 ms after the triggering spike. Where there are multiple potentials of extraordinary length, the sweep speed should be adjusted accordingly, with the aid of acoustical monitoring. At least 20 estimations should be made from different recording sites with at least four separate skin penetrations.

It is essential that one of the components be made maximal, i.e. one fibre must be approached as closely as possible by the recording electrode when the other components are to be counted. This is in contrast to the technique for recording the jitter, in which the electrode position is adjusted to record from two muscle fibres with optimal amplitudes. Theoretically, two fibres can be as much as 400 μm apart and still fulfil the criteria if the recording electrode lies between them. This is acceptable for jitter calculations, but for fibre density measurement only one of these

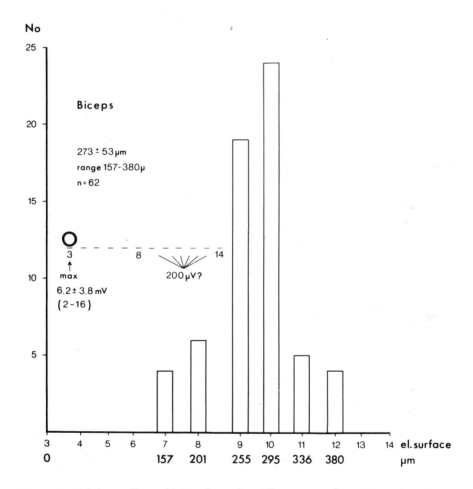

Fig. 34   Uptake radius of the electrode. The outer electrode surface in the multi-electrode is positioned close to the studied muscle fibre. The electrode surface at which the action potential is reduced most closely to 200 μV is identified. The mean distance from this surface to the reference electrode is approximately the same as to the muscle fibre and therefore equals the uptake radius of the electrode for the given criteria. The recordings were made in the biceps brachii muscle.

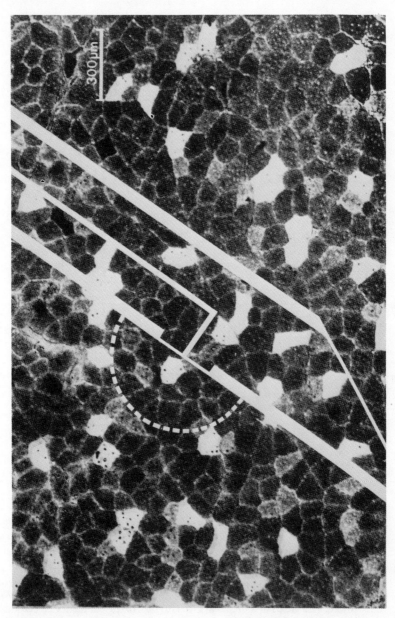

Fig. 35   Cross-section of muscle stained for glycogen after stimulating an isolated motor axon to show one motor unit (From Edström and Kugelberg, 1968). An SFEMG electrode is superimposed to show the uptake area.

fibres should be recorded if the electrode has been correctly approximated to it (Fig. 36). When moving to the next site, the electrode should be advanced enough to lose all previously recorded potentials.

Normal Fibre Density

There are slight differences in normal fibre density in different muscles (Table 5). In normal adults fibre density in the biceps brachii is slightly lower, and in the frontalis higher, than in most other muscles. In the normal extensor digitorum communis muscle, single fibres from individual motor units are recorded in 65–70% of random insertions, two fibres in about 30% and 3 or 4 fibres seldom[57]. This corresponds to an average of 1.5 fibres per uptake area of the electrode. The fibre density is normally slightly higher under the age of 10 years, and increases again over the age of 60 years (Fig. 37). The increase in fibre density with advancing years, most pronounced in tibialis anterior and extensor digitorum brevis, is supposed to be a result of compensatory reinnervation associated with normal neuronal fall-out.

The reason for the slightly higher fibre density in young children is not yet clear. One possibility is that smaller fibre diameters result in a large number of fibres per unit of cross-sectional area. The effect of such "packing" of fibres on the fibre density should be to some extent counteracted by the smaller electrical fields of individual fibres, and therefore the smaller uptake area of the electrode. Other possible explanations include different volume conduction characteristics of the muscle tissue, or different arrangements of muscle fibres in motor unit territory in the young.

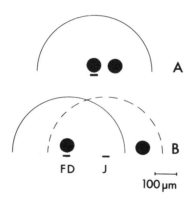

Fig. 36   Different recording positions for fibre density and jitter measurements. For fibre density measurement the electrode must be as close as possible to one active muscle fibre, indicated in A and as FD position in B. In B only one fibre is then recorded. In jitter measurements the electrode position is adjusted to obtain recordings from potential pairs. This is achieved in A with the same position as for fibre density measurement but in B another position must be used (J). If this position were used for fibre density measurement the value would be erroneously high. Semicircles indicate the uptake area of the electrode.

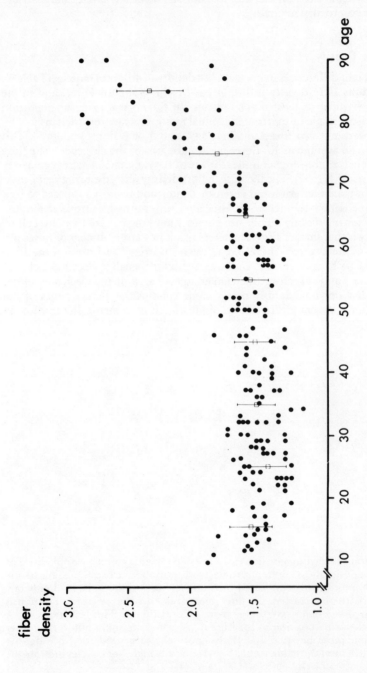

Fig. 37   Fibre density values in EDC in different ages. Each dot represents the mean number of muscle fibres/uptake area of the electrode belonging to the same motor unit in one subject. Mean values and standard deviations for each decade are indicated (From Thiele and Stålberg, 1975).

AGES

Muscles	10–25 years			26–50 years			51–75 years			above 75 years		
	m	SD	n	m	SD	n	m	SD	n	m	SD	n
Frontalis	1.61	0.21	(11)	1.72	0.21	(15)						
Deltoid	1.36	0.16	(20)	1.40	0.11	(10)						
Biceps	1.25	0.09	(20)	1.33	0.07	(17)						
Extensor digitorum communis	1.47	0.16	(61)	1.49	0.16	(98)	1.57	0.17	(59)	2.13	0.41	(21)
1st dorsal interosseus	1.33	0.13	(14)	1.45	0.12	(6)						
Rectus femoris	1.43	0.18	(11)	1.57	0.23	(14)						
Tibialis anterior	1.57	0.22	(18)	1.56	0.22	(21)	1.77	0.12	(4)			
Extensor digitorum brevis	2.07	0.42	(16)	2.62	0.30	(11)				3.8		(1)

Table 5. Fibre density in different muscles of normal subjects arranged in four age groups. Number of subjects (n) in parentheses.

Abnormal Fibre Density

After reinnervation the fibre density is increased owing to collateral sprouting, and 3–10 fibres from the same motor unit may often be recorded at an electrode position (Fig. 38); increased fibre density does indeed usually indicate collateral sprouting[54]. There is a correlation between histochemical fibre-type grouping and increased fibre density. The fibre density value is however a more sensitive index, showing slight rearrangements within the motor unit even before fibre-type grouping is evident. Another cause, general muscle atrophy with shrinkage, has been considered, but this should decrease the amplitude of the volume conducted spikes and, using the criteria given, the uptake area of the electrode. Selective atrophy with shrinkage of motor units of one or the other type might cause condensation of other motor units and thus an increase in the fibre density per area unit. This possible cause of increase in fibre density has to be further investigated. Splitting of fibres, particularly seen in muscular dystrophies may also increase fibre density (page 148). It should be noted that a drop-out of fibres within the motor unit is generally not detected. The lowest possible value is 1.0, which is inherent in the technique. As soon as there is a tendency to clustering of fibres within the motor unit, the fibre density value is increased. It is not a measure of the total number of fibres in a motor unit, but of the average number of fibres within the pick-up area of the electrode wherever there is at least one fibre belonging to that unit. It is thus an index of the local concentration of action potential generators activated from the same motor unit, which would include muscle fibres, fibre branches and, hypothetically, even muscle fibres belonging to other units but being driven ephaptically by muscle fibres of the unit under consideration.

DURATION OF MULTIPLE POTENTIALS

The duration of a recorded action potential complex is measured from the zero intersection line of the first action potential fulfilling the recording criteria (of 200 μV amplitude and a rise time of less than 300 μs) to the zero intersection line of the last component. For the normal EDC muscle this value is below 4 ms in over 95%. The chance of recording longer complexes increases with insertions far outside the motor end-plate zone. It is also higher in the frontalis and brachioradialis (see page 27).

Another useful parameter is the *mean interspike interval (MISI)*, i.e. the total duration divided by the number of intervals, or, number of components minus one. This is increased particularly in muscular dystrophies and polymyositis and usually in early reinnervation. The normal range of MISI in the extensor digitorum communis is 0.3–0.7 ms (table 6). The duration of a multiple action potential depends on the difference in conduction times in the nerve branches, motor end-plates and muscle fibres taken by the impulses which generate the various spike components.

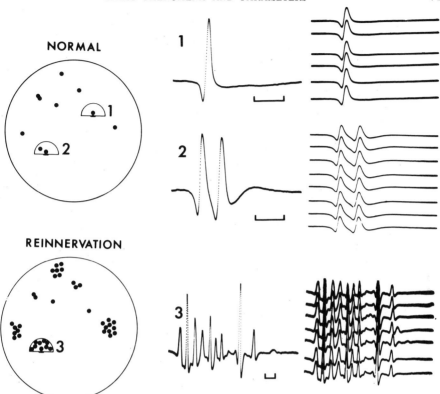

Fig. 38 Single Fibre EMG recordings in normal and reinnervated muscle. The diagram illustrates the number of muscle fibres of one motor unit (blackened). The uptake area of the recording electrode is represented as half circle. In the normal (1 and 2) only action potentials from one or two fibres are recorded. In reinnervation (3) many fibre action potentials are recorded due to increased fibre density in the motor unit. (Time cal 1 ms)

MUSCLES	MISI		
	Mean	SD	n
Frontalis	1.02	0.29	(22)
Deltoid	0.46	0.17	(25)
Biceps	0.42	0.18	(17)
Extensor digitorum communis	0.64	0.30	(46)
1st dorsal interosseus	0.42	0.18	(19)
Rectus femoris	0.60	0.34	(23)
Tibialis anterior	0.52	0.13	(19)
Extensor digitorum brevis	0.53	0.14	(26)

Table 6.   Mean interspike interval values in muscles of normal subjects aged 10 to 75 years.

PROPAGATION VELOCITY AND DIRECTION
OF PROPAGATION

Recording Procedure

For measuring the propagation velocity[42] a multi-electrode recording is required, such as an electrode with two arrays of recording surfaces, 1 + 13 (Fig. 4), connected to two amplifiers. An electrode position is sought in which on one channel a single fibre action potential is optimally recorded from the single electrode placed opposite to the long row a few hundred μm from its centre. To the other amplifier system the electrodes in the long row are successively connected, and the electrode that records the action potential with the largest amplitude is chosen for measurement. The multi-electrode is now rotated until the same action potential amplitude is obtained from the two electrodes. Minor to and fro movements of the electrode are then performed until a position is reached at which the amplitudes of the two action potentials decrease and increase in parallel. At this correct electrode position there is a small difference between the two recorded action potentials due to cross-talk between the leads in the shaft and, to a minor degree, in other parts of the recording system. The negative peak of the first action potential and the positive peak of the second are slightly rounded and reduced in amplitude. Otherwise the potentials should be identical, with their steep deflections parallel (Fig. 39).

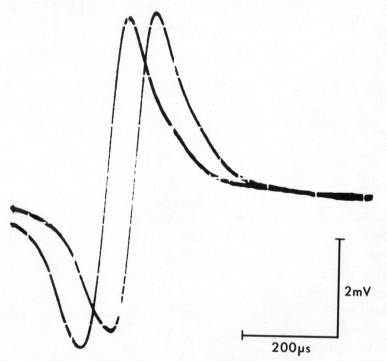

Fig. 39   Single fibre action potential recorded from two electrode surfaces in a multi-electrode 200 μm apart.

When an optimal recording position has been achieved, the time between the two recorded potentials is measured with an electronic time counter at corresponding points close to the zero intersection point. The time resolution should be 0.1 μs. A jitter in interpotential time exceeding 5 μs between the two potentials indicates that the two electrodes are recording activity from two different muscle fibres. This recording cannot be used for propagation velocity measurements. By dividing the inter-electrode distance, known from microphotographs, by the recorded time interval, the propagation velocity across the electrode is obtained. The possible inaccuracy of the electrode position may introduce an error (overestimation) in the length of distance travelled along the muscle fibre of less than 5%. The time measurement is made with an accuracy of ±1μs which may result in an error in propagation velocity estimation of less than 1%. The direction of impulse transmission across the multi-electrode can be determined from the propagation velocity recording, from which it is immediately possible to detect which of the two electrodes receives the impulse first. In this way, the localisation of the motor end-plate in relation to the recording site can be determined. By making multiple determinations of the propagation direction at each of many levels along the muscle between the two tendons the motor end-plate zone can be mapped, particularly in muscles with one main fibre orientation.

Normal Values

The range of normal muscle fibre propagation velocity values lies between 1.5 and 6.5 m/s but varies from muscle to muscle and even within a given muscle (Table 7). Experiments on isolated muscle fibres (Håkansson 1956) have shown that one of the factors determining the propagation velocity is the muscle fibre diameter. This is exemplified by the findings in a patient in whom the propagation velocity in a quadriceps muscle with disuse atrophy after an operation on the patella was 2.8 ± 0.4 m/s, compared with 3.5 ± 0.7 m/s in the normal quadriceps (P < 0.01). Propagation velocity values can, in fact, be used as a relative measure of muscle fibre diameter distribution in all muscles on which EMG can be performed. Low propagation

MUSCLE	NUMBER OF FIBRES	PROPAGATION VELOCITY (M/S)	
		MEAN	SD
Biceps brachii	443	3.7	0.7
Extensor digitorum communis	161	3.2	0.8
Quadriceps femoris	142	3.4	0.7
Frontalis	26	2.0	0.4

Table 7. Propagation velocity in different muscles.

velocity values are found in neurogenic atrophy, particularly for late components of multiple action potentials, and also in muscular dystrophies (page 141). Different correlation factors between muscle fibre diameter and propagation velocity have, it is true, been reported by different authors, and it should be noted that the diameter-velocity correlation has been determined in normal muscle fibres in vitro. The correlation coefficient may be different in pathological situations, with altered membrane characteristics and perhaps changed electrolyte balance.

Propagation Velocity During Continuous Activity

During continued activation the propagation velocity usually decreases most during the first minute.[42] The decrease in velocity can amount to 50% of the inital value over a period of 3 minutes (Fig. 40). When a pause is introduced, the propagation velocity recovers to a degree depending on the length of the pause. This decrease in propagation velocity might explain the change in power spectrum with the concentric needle EMG when the higher frequencies decrease and low frequencies increase during continuous activity. A special method for analysing the surface EMG (Lindström, 1970) provides an indirect measure of the mean propagation velocity in the muscle and demonstrates a decrease during continuous activity.

Interdischarge Interval-dependent Variability: the Velocity Recovery Function (VRF)

The propagation velocity values for consecutive impulses show a slight variability which depends strictly on the previous impulse interval[42]. A short interval after the preceding discharge is followed by an increased propagation velocity, though this does not hold true for extremely short intervals, such as in extra-discharges. The phenomenon can be studied in detail with double pulse stimulation. A subnormal propagation velocity is seen for a test impulse after an interval of 3–10 ms, with a reduction by 20% for the shortest intervals. A supernormal velocity is found at intervals between 10 and 1000 ms with maximum at about 50 ms. The propagation velocity can here be increased by 10–15% relative to the conditioning impulse (Fig. 41). This velocity recovery function (VRF) depends on the restoration of the membrane potential after the passage of an impulse and probably reflects other membrane characteristics than those responsible for the propagation velocity value itself, which is mainly correlated to the fibre diameter. The remaining VRF effect for each impulse is added to the next and at physiological innervation rates the propagation velocity in the single fibre is always influenced by previous activity. The VRF can be studied with double pulse stimulation and is found to be approximately exponential for intervals exceeding 30 ms. For intervals from 30–1000 ms (the supernormal part of the curve) data are more easily obtained from the voluntarily activated muscle, with the discharge pattern being made irregular to produce variable interdischarge intervals. By means of computer analysis the VRF of a muscle fibre can be plotted from velocity values obtained at irregular innervation rates. It is not possible to calculate the VRF directly from the ratio between propagation velocity and the preceding interdischarge interval, since the change in propagation velocity for a given interval is determined by the propagation velocity value in the preceding

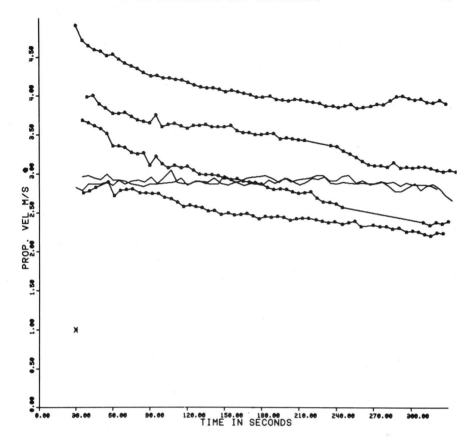

Fig. 40   Decrease of propagation velocity in four muscle fibres during continued
activity at 11, 16, 12 and 9 discharges/s respectively (asterisks). In a fifth
fibre, tested at an innervation rate of 6 and 16 discharges/s (the two full
lines) there is no decrease in propagation velocity.

(reference) discharge (Fig. 41). Therefore the propagation velocity values for a series
of discharges with non-uniform intervals has to be subdivided into velocity classes
(class width 0.1 m/s). Now each propagation velocity value within the individual class
is considered as a reference value and the succeeding propagation velocity value is
plotted against the interdischarge interval. A family of curves is thus obtained (Fig.
42), each with different steepness (steeper for higher reference values) but
representing the same exponential function, i.e. the relative decrease for a given
interval is the same. The relative decrease of the supernormality in intervals between
50–100 ms has been chosen to express the slope of the curve. This slope differs for
different fibres and has been used in some investigations as a quantitative parameter
to classify the VRF into 4 categories: a decrease of 0–10% = "no VRF",
10–20% = slight, 20–30% = moderate, more than 30% = pronounced VRF. Excep-

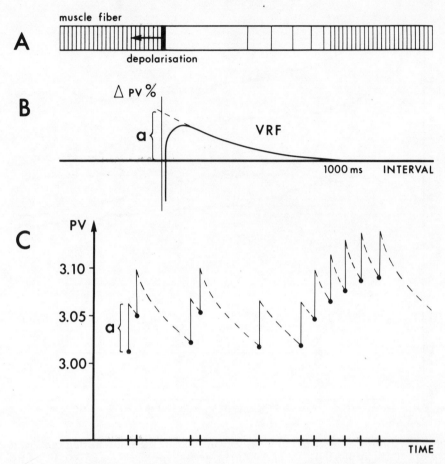

Fig.41   Propagation velocity recovery function (VRF) in a muscle fibre. Immediately after the passage of an impulse the muscle fibre is refractory, after which it propagates a succeeding impulse first at subnormal and then at supernormal velocity (A). This change in propagation velocity can be tested with double pulse stimulation (B). The increment varies typically between 0 and 15% in the normal muscle. The remaining effect of preceding impulses is added to subsequent impulses, and at irregular activation rate (C) the propagation velocity for successive discharge varies.

tional fibres with a long subnormal phase without supernormality are classified as "negative". Examples are shown in Fig. 43.

The supernormal velocity is found in about 50–70% of normal muscle fibres studied. Normally, there are no fibres showing only a long subnormal phase but this happens often at low temperature and during ischaemia when the positive VRF disappears. In muscular dystrophies the positive VRF is present in a higher proportion of all fibres[44], and when present it is also more pronounced (page 141).

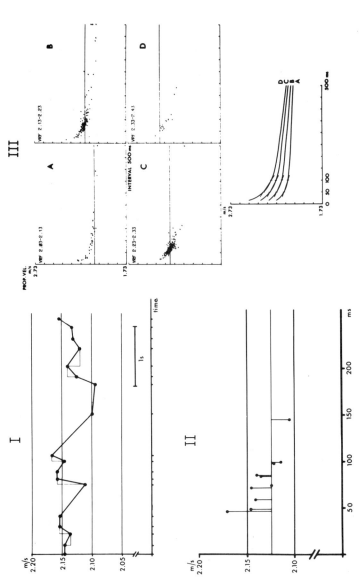

Fig. 42   Principles for the analysis of the velocity recovery function at voluntary innervation. The propagation velocity values are divided into classes. In I the values between propagation velocity 2.10 and 2.15 m/s are thus analysed. All action potentials with propagation velocity within a certain class are considered as conditioning impulses. The change in propagation velocity to the next action potential, the test impulse, is calculated as well as the time interval to this. For each class the change for the test impulse propagation velocity (ordinate) is plotted against the time interval from the conditioning impulse (abscissa) as made in II. The time scale is different in I and II. In III, a computer printout for another fibre with data in four different classes is shown.

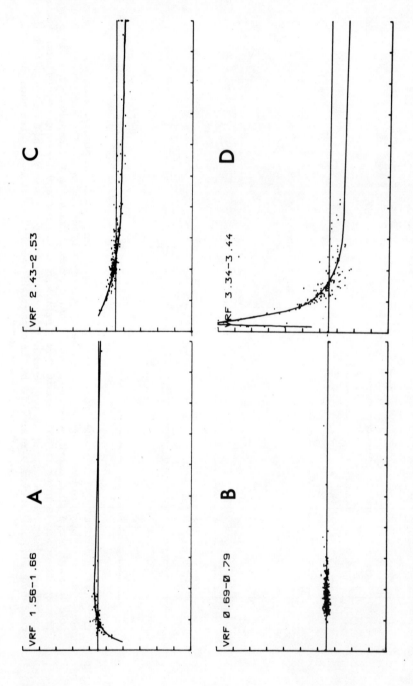

Fig. 43   Examples of computer printouts of VRF curves of four different fibres. A = negative, B = "no VRF", C = slight and D = pronounced VRF. The recordings are randomly taken from myotonic dystrophy, distal myopathy and limb-girdle dystrophy. (From Stålberg, 1977)

DISCHARGE CHARACTERISTICS

Firing Pattern

The recruitment order and firing patterns of motor units have been studied by many authors. In general the recruitment order is relatively fixed during gradually increasing strength. The low threshold units have smaller ventral horn cells, smaller axons and contain smaller and perhaps also fewer muscle fibres. The recruitment order can be slightly changed if the movement is initiated in a phasic manner or under certain experimental conditions (Hannerz and Grimby, 1973). Attempts have been made to use the firing pattern to separate tonic from phasic motor units. One of the most commonly used measures has been the variability of the instant rate at different mean frequencies. Tokizane and Shimazu (1964) found two populations of motor units, one low-threshold with a relatively constant firing rate even at low mean frequencies, and another one recruited at higher strengths and showing a more irregular firing pattern. The two populations were referred to as tonic and kinetic units, respectively. These findings could not be reproduced by other authors (Milner-Brown, Stein and Yemm, 1973c; Petajan and Phillip, 1969), nor in our own study.

We have studied the firing pattern mainly of those motor units recruited with low to moderate effort, usually at less than 30% of maximal force[56]. Individual motor units have a lowest preferred rate of firing which differs for different muscles (5 discharges/s for back muscles and quadriceps femoris, 7-9 for biceps brachii). If the subject is asked to produce 5 discharges/s of a motor unit with a lowest preferred rate of 7 the activity will consist of a few discharges with a mean rate of 7, separated by pauses which make the mean rate of 5 per second over a longer period. With increasing strength the mean rate increases and the pattern becomes more regular. For proper analysis of the mean rate versus its variability (SD or coefficient of variation) slow trends have to be subtracted. This can be done by calculating a sliding mean over, for example, 9 data and subtracting this value from the middle datum in each set (i.e. No. 5). The sliding mean is probably influenced by other factors such as afferent input during breathing.

In studies of firing patterns in which subjects were instructed to keep desired firing rates constant at different levels, clear inter-individual differences were found in the ability to do this. Within the same muscle a great variation between different motor units has been observed, but no significant bimodal distribution detected. One reason may be that mostly tonic units have been studied even though higher activation strengths have been used. The highest continued innervation rate obtained has been about 30 discharges/s, but for short phasic contractions rates as high as 75 have been reported (Hannerz, 1975).

There is no evidence for a rotation of activity within the motor unit or between different motor units in a continuously contracting muscle. Statistical analysis of multi-unit recordings has not shown that synchrony occurs between the firing of different motor units in the normal rested muscle, at slight or moderate effort. During a great effort, and especially during fatigue, there is a tendency for motor units to fire synchronously.

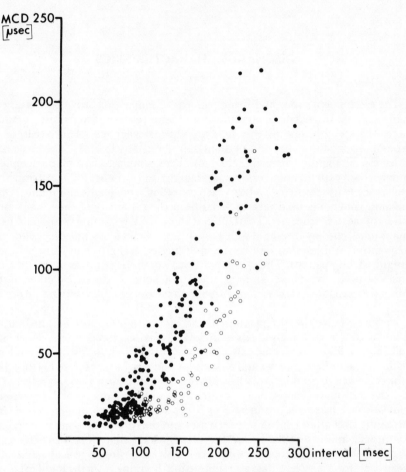

Fig. 44   Interdischarge interval irregularity of motoneurones from the m. extensor digitorum communis (●) and the m. longissimus dorsi (o). Abscissa: mean interval. Ordinate: interval irregularity measured as MCD: Each motoneurone is represented by 3–10 points having a characteristic local distribution in the material. No separation in two types of motoneurone occurred in each muscle, but the two muscles show different distributions. The limit frequencies for extensor digitorum communis motoneurones were typically 8–10/s and for the lumbar muscle 5–7/s causing a shift to the right for the interval-MCD curve of the latter (From Stålberg and Thiele, 1973).

Extra-Discharges

An extra firing of the motor unit being studied may occasionally be seen a short time (4–15 ms) after the original discharge. The extra-discharge is identified by: the similarity in its shape to that of the original action potential, the variation of its

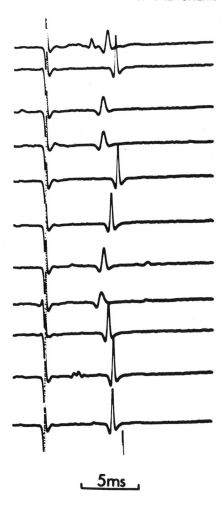

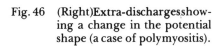

Fig. 45 (Above) Extra-discharges with pronounced change in amplitude and rise time at intervals below 5 ms (in a case of Duchenne dystrophy).

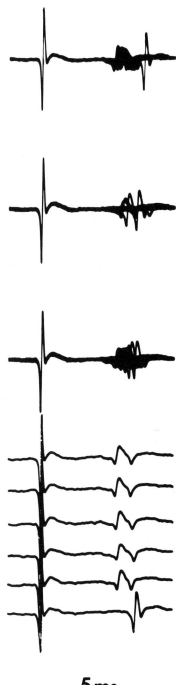

Fig. 46 (Right) Extra-discharges showing a change in the potential shape (a case of polymyositis).

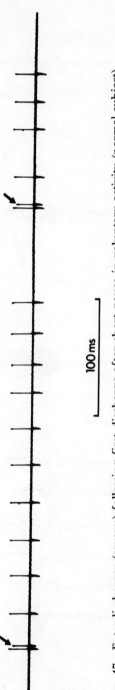

Fig. 47   Extradischarges (arrows) following first discharge after short pause in voluntary activity (normal subject).

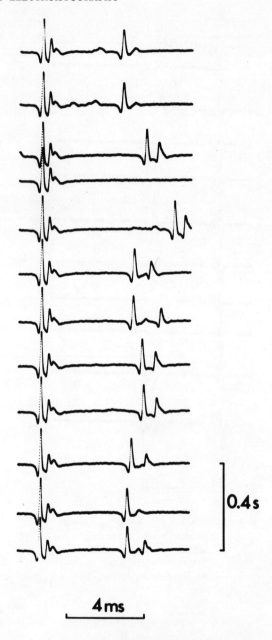

Fig. 48   Extra-discharge of a potential pair showing increase in interspike interval and blocking of the second potential at the shortest interval.

amplitude in parallel with the original potential on electrode movement, and a progressive reduction in amplitude when the interval to the extra-discharge is shorter than 10 ms (Fig. 45); thus there is a reduction by up to 25–30% for a 5 ms interval, and by 75% for a 4 ms interval. The total duration is prolonged, the rise time at the shortest intervals being up to 3 times longer than in the original discharge. In this case the biphasic shape may be changed to triphasic and even "disintegrate" (Fig. 46).

In the normal muscle the extra-discharge is particularly likely to follow the first discharge when voluntary activity is resumed after a pause (Fig. 47). The interval to the extra-discharge is usually between 15 and 30 ms, and the interval to the next normal discharge is not influenced. This type of extra-discharge is believed to be centrally generated, and is not found to be correlated to any pathology.

In pathological conditions the successive intervals between the original and the extra-discharge may be quite stable (less than 0.5 ms range), particularly in motor neurone disorders,[54] or vary by as much as 5 ms or more, as is commonly seen in tetany,[76] muscular dystrophies[44] and polymyositis. When the potential has multiple spikes, the extra-discharge usually contains all the original components. The intervals between the individual spike components and their shape and amplitude are usually slightly changed in the extra-discharge due to sub- or supernormality of the nerve and muscle fibres at this short interval after the original discharge. Also, one or more individual components may be missing in the extra-discharge (Fig. 48).

In cases of muscular dystrophy it is sometimes also possible to observe the reverse phenomenon, the recruitment of additional components due to facilitation,[44] which should not be mistaken for an extra-discharge. The order of invidual components may exceptionally be reversed in the extra-discharge, which may be due to very peripheral generation (Fig. 49). When the appearance of the extra-discharge changes for any of these reasons its true nature may not be immediately recognized, and it may be misinterpreted as a blocking part of a multispike potential (Fig. 48). In some cases the extra-discharges appear above or below certain innervation rates and can then regularly follow every discharge.

Sometimes, particularly in dystrophia myotonica, the extra-discharge prevents the occurrence of the following regular discharge, resulting in doubling of the original inter-discharge interval. This is probably a peripheral phenomenon, due to prolonged refractoriness of a weak point in the nerve fibre, perhaps identical with the one at which the extra-discharges are being generated.

Fasciculations

Fasciculation potentials recorded by SFEMG usually appear as multispike discharges occurring at irregular intervals. In normal muscle they are as a rule very stable, of constant shape and with normal or low jitter between individual spike components at repetitive discharges (Fig. 50 A and B). This type may also be seen in pathological conditions of the lower motor neurone but it is more usual, in amyotrophic lateral sclerosis for example, to record increased jitter, intermittent blocking and, less commonly, a changing spike order[54] (Fig. 50 C).

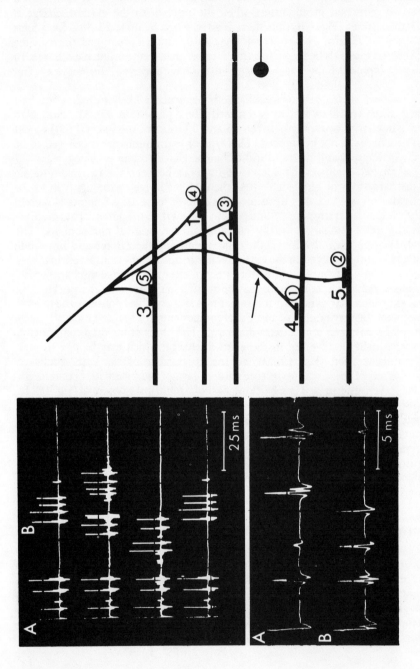

Fig. 49 An example of extradischarges of a multiple spike potential in Duchenne dystrophy. Notice that the order of individual spikes is different in the extradischarges (B, circles in the drawing) from that in the original discharges (A). (From Stålberg, 1977)

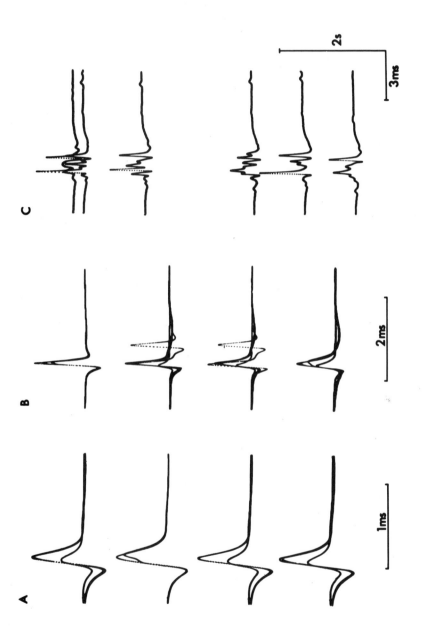

Fig. 50 Fasciculation potentials. A and B, in a normal subject. Superimpositions of 5 successive discharges occurring at a rate of about 2 per minute. Number of muscle fibres participating varies, their action potentials are frequently superimposed on each other, jitter is normal or low. C, a sequence of irregularly occurring variable multi-spike discharges with increased jitter between the individual components, in a case of long-standing poliomyelitis with recent deterioration. Note a double discharge (uppermost pair of traces).

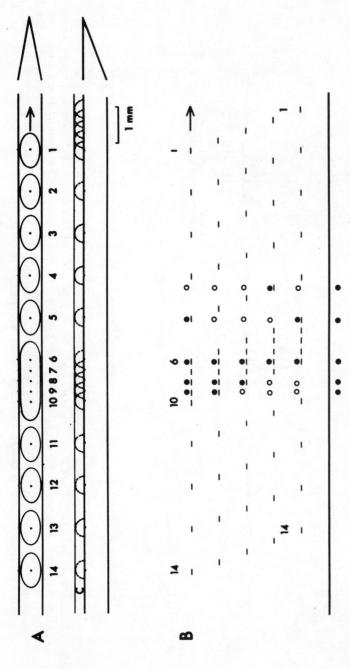

Fig. 51   A. The multi-electrode used for the study of the motor unit. In the side view the uptake area of the individual electrode surfaces (dotted semi-circles) and the recording corridor (C) are indicated. For electrode surface 1 the effect of completed movement in the study of one corridor is shown.

B. The principle of the multi-electrode movements allowing recording from 45 sites, 300 μm apart. Only the electrode surfaces are indicated. The electrode arrays for each step are drawn below each other although the 4 advancements are in one and the same corridor along the multi-electrode axis. Top row: initial position with "reference action potential" over electrode 6. Responses are obtained over electrodes 5, 8 and 9. The electrode is then advanced 300 μm so that electrode 7 becomes the reference electrode and responses are recorded over electrodes 9 and 10. At next two advancements (with reference electrodes 8 and 9) only 2 responses are obtained. At the last movement the response originally obtained from electrode 5 is obtained at electrode 6, which is a proof of correctly completed study. The distribution of the motor unit's muscle fibres in the corridor after the four movements covering the complete length is indicated at the bottom.

MULTI-ELECTRODE STUDIES

In order to study the distribution of the muscle fibres in the motor unit, a multi-electrode technique has been devised.[53] The multi-electrode consists of a steel cannula 0.6 mm in diameter with 14 platinum electrode surfaces 25 μm in diameter arranged over a total distance of 12 mm. The inter-electrode distance between electrodes 1–6 and 10–14 is approximately 1.2 mm, and the inter-electrode distance for the central electrodes 6 to 10 is approximately 0.3 mm. Thus the total distance between electrodes 6 and 10 is similar to the larger inter-electrode distance (Fig. 51 A). The recordings are made simultaneously from two of the electrodes against a cutaneous indifferent electrode.

RECORDING PROCEDURE

The multi-electrode is inserted perpendicularly to the muscle fibres. To begin with, recording is made from electrode 6, which is the first "reference electrode". The multi-electrode is then positioned to obtain a single fibre action potential of high amplitude and short rise time. This "reference action potential" is displayed on the first beam of the oscilloscope and triggers the sweep. The electrode position is maintained and recordings are made successively from the other electrode surfaces by means of automatic or manual electronic switching after 10 or 20 discharges of the triggering potential. The activity from the other electrodes is displayed on the second beam. The presence of action potentials time-locked to the triggering one, i.e. activity from fibres belonging to the same motor unit, is noted for each of the electrodes. Delay lines (5 ms) are used for both of the recording channels to identify action potentials occurring before the triggering one. In order to be accepted, the action potential must reach an amplitude greater than 200 μV, have a fast rise time (less than 300 μs) and be seen on consecutive discharges. According to these criteria only single fibre action potentials relatively near, (250–300 μm, page 64) to the active recording electrodes are counted. Muscle fibres close to one electrode are usually recorded with an amplitude of less than 200 μV at the next recording position, 300 μm away. However, a muscle fibre situated between two recording positions 300 μm apart may fulfil the criteria for acceptance at both electrodes. In order to test if the two action potentials are generated by one or two muscle fibres, recording is made from both surfaces simultaneously and the time relation between the potentials is studied. The presence of a jitter between them indicates recording from two fibres.[47] If there is no jitter at successive discharges the recordings are obtained from the same muscle fibre. When the same muscle fibre action potential is picked up at two or more recording sites 300 μm apart it is only counted once, at the electrode at which the amplitude is highest (Fig. 52).

With one position of the multi-electrode, the potentials arising from some fibres belonging to the same motor unit within the uptake corridor will not appear at any of the 13 other electrodes, owing to the long inter-electrode distances (1.2 mm) of electrodes 1–6 and 10–14, so the multi-electrode is advanced 300 μm until the

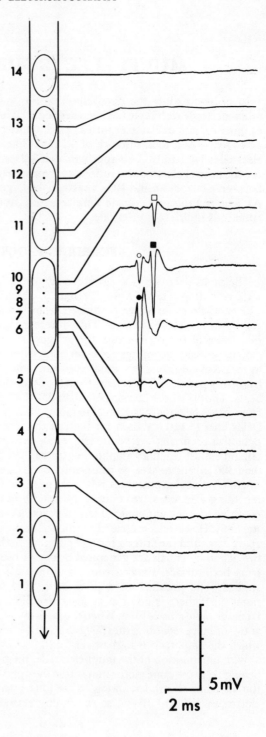

Fig. 52   The multi-electrode, with 14 platinum 25 μm recording surfaces. The action potentials recorded at one position are shown on the right. Two of the action potentials are each recorded from two electrodes (8–9, circles and 9–10 squares) but the responses are only counted when they appear with maximal amplitude (8 and 9). A third action potential (asterix) fulfilling the criteria for acceptance is seen over electrode 7.
(From Stålberg, Schwartz, Thiele and Schiller, 1976)

"reference action potential" is recorded over electrode 7 with the same shape as it had over electrode 6. This is made easier by the simultaneous display of activity at both the new and the former reference electrode while advancing the multi-electrode. All other electrodes are then rescanned. The multi-electrode is advanced in steps of 300 μm so that the "reference action potential" is picked up successively by electrodes 8, 9 and 10. In this way all fibres along the entire recording corridor can be identified (Fig. 51·B).

When the "reference action potential" has been advanced from electrode 6 to electrode 10 the electrode is moved 1.2 mm, which exactly corresponds to the inter-electrode distances for the spaced electrodes. Thus if responses were initially obtained over electrodes 2, 5 and 6 the same responses should, after the completed manoeuvre, be recorded over electrodes 3, 6 and 10. This constancy confirms that electrode movements have been correct, and is the usual finding in these investigations. Should the response profile change after a full advancement, that recording is discarded. In about a third of the trials the procedure could not be completed owing to the loss of the "reference action potential". If no responses are obtained apart from the "reference action potential", so that it is impossible to monitor the response profile, characteristics such as shape and firing pattern are used to identify this action potential on successive electrode movements. It is much easier to follow the "reference action potential" when it is complex. The investigation of an individual motor unit takes 5–10 minutes and subsequent analysis is made from the analogue magnetic tape.

The Uptake Area of the Electrode

The total leading-off area of this electrode is somewhat complex. Since the 5 central electrodes have an intercentre distance of 300 μm their uptake areas overlap. When the electrode has been advanced successively over the four 300 μm steps the recorded "corridor" consists of 45 hemispheres, each with an uptake radius of about 300 μm and an intercentre distance of 300 μm, corresponding to a total length of 13.8 mm ($46 \times 0.3 = 13.8$). There is a slight "dead space" in the corridor of about 15% due to the hemispherical uptake area of each recording surface (Fig. 51 A).

THE MOTOR UNIT IN NORMAL MUSCLE

The multi-electrode technique has been used to map the fibre arrangement in the normal motor unit.[53] The distribution of fibres within single corridors in the EDC muscle is seen in Fig. 53. The average number of fibres over the reference electrode was 1.4; SD 0.2 in EDC and 1.3; SD 0.2 in the biceps brachii muscle. For the other electrodes the fibre density over the electrode at which potentials were recorded was 1.2 in EDC and 1.2 in the biceps brachii muscle.

There were no definite differences relative to age from 20 to 70 years. In the individual corridor 1 to 9 fibres were seen both in EDC and in biceps brachii. Nine fibres were seen in three of the 101 recordings from 2 muscles. The range of mean values of the number of fibres in the recorded corridors was from 2.5 to 4.9 (mean 3.9; SD 0.8) in EDC and 1.9 to 5.5 (mean 3.7; SD 1.3) in the biceps brachii. In EDC there were 13 recordings in which action potentials were picked up by only the

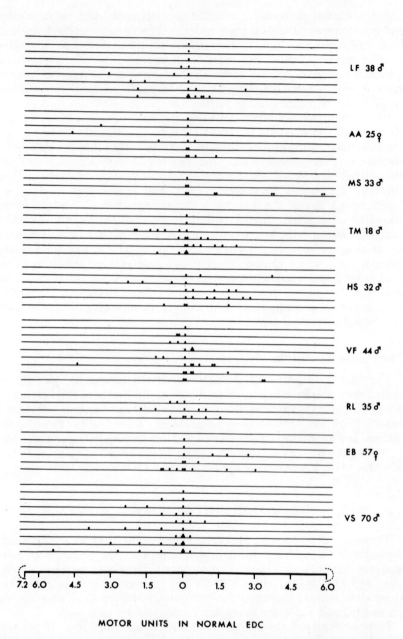

MOTOR UNITS IN NORMAL EDC

Fig. 53 Motor unit corridors in normal extensor digitorum communis muscles. Each dot represents a different single muscle fibre. The initial reference electrode (6) is at distance 0.
(From Stålberg, Schwartz, Thiele and Schiller, 1976)

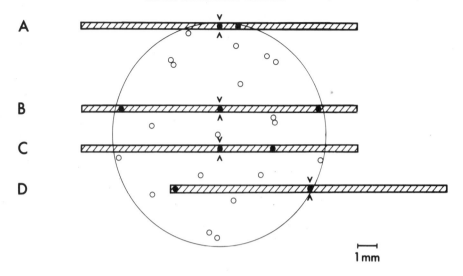

RECORDING CORRIDOR OF THE MULTIELECTRODE

Fig. 54   Maximal distance between responses in the recording corridor of the multi-electrode. Only in B is the diameter of the "motor unit territory" estimated appropriately. Peripherally running corridor (A), missing borderline fibres (C) and asymmetric probing (D) are factors causing underestimation of the "motor unit territory". Ⅴ indicates the reference electrode.

reference electrode (24%) and in biceps brachii also 13 recordings showed no additional fibres (27%).

When the "reference action potential" was a single fibre action potential there was for EDC an average of 2.1 fibres outside the reference electrode, for double spikes an average of 2.9 additional fibres, and for 3 reference action potentials another 3.4 fibres were recorded. The corresponding figures for biceps were 1.9, 3.5 and 5 (one case), respectively. Even though the number of additional fibres was increased in the corridor when the "reference action potential" was complex, the fibre density over active electrodes was not similarly increased. In none of the 101 corridors studied were there more than 3 fibres over any electrode.

"Motor Unit Territory"

The longest distance between two fibres recorded in a single motor unit study was 6 mm (three recordings) in EDC and 6–7 mm (five recordings) and 9 mm (one recording) in biceps brachii. While maximal inter-fibre distance may give some information about the motor unit territory, these measurements should not be taken to indicate that the method is suitable for its precise delineation (Fig. 54). This is due to the dimensions of the recording area, which measures 13.8 × 0.270 mm. Although the length of the electrode is appropriate (other studies having indicated that motor unit territories are generally less than 10 mm) the narrowness of the recording corridor will introduce errors, since there is a considerable risk that muscle fibres at the border of the motor unit will be missed. Moreover, many corridors will obviously not run through the centre of the motor units and the diameters will be underestimated. It may nevertheless be that where motor units are very dense after collateral sprouting the extreme inter-fibre distances at the periphery may be a more accurate guide to the anatomical size of the motor unit than they are in normal muscle.

Comments on Multi-electrode Findings in Normal Muscle

This study has shown that in the normal human EDC and biceps muscles the muscle fibres of a single motor unit are scattered in a way similar to that already demonstrated in animals by means of glycogen depletion experiments (Edström and Kugelberg, 1968; Brandstater and Lambert, 1969; Doyle and Mayer, 1969). A single motor unit's distribution covers about 17% of the cross-sectional area of the rat tibialis anterior muscle (Kugelberg, 1973). In such studies it has been found that in rats the fibres of a single motor unit are usually isolated; 76% of the fibres are not adjacent to any other fibre of the same motor unit, and only rarely are three fibres found together (Brandstater and Lambert, 1969). These figures are comparable to the fibre density values obtained with single fibre EMG in human muscles in which an isolated fibre is recorded in 60–65% of random electrode placements. We have not found more than three fibres over one leading-off surface out of 300 active electrodes used in the study of 101 normal motor units. This accords with the results of conventional histochemistry; thus the mosaic pattern of fibre-type distribution in a cross-sectional area of muscle in man (Engel, 1966; Jennekens, Tomlinson and Walton, 1971) indicated scattering, though the method could not identify the individual motor units, and in a single case of myokymia glycogen-depleted fibres of one or more active units were randomly scattered (Williamsson and Brooke, 1972). In conclusion, multi-electrode investigations have demonstrated how muscle fibres in individual motor units are distributed in the normal EDC and biceps brachii muscle. The fibres were found to be dispersed in a manner similar to that shown in the experimental glycogen-depletion studies. Some motor units seem to be generally denser than others.

PHARMACOLOGICAL STUDIES OF NEUROMUSCULAR TRANSMISSION

ANTI-DEPOLARIZING AGENTS

Conventional studies of neuromuscular transmission in man are at present based upon the supramaximal electrical stimulation of a motor nerve and the measurement of either the mechanical response of the muscle or the amplitude of the compound action potential generated by the muscle. By this means it is possible to estimate the percentage of motor end-plates developing total block as a result of the action of a blocking agent tested during the course of repetitive stimulation. Much earlier, even subclinical, interference with neuromuscular transmission may be observed by means of a jitter study in voluntarily or electrically activated muscle.[14, 45] Typical findings are as follows:

A systemic injection of 15 μg d-Tubocurarine per kg body weight leads to a slight increase in jitter, by 5–15 μs. After a dose of 30 μg/kg the effect is more pronounced and the jitter increases by up to 20 μs; it begins to increase at 20–30 seconds after injection, reaches a peak after 2–5 minutes and declines slowly in the next 10–30 minutes. When higher doses are used, occasional blocking of either potential of a pair tends to occur when the jitter exceeds 70 to 80 μs.[35] With a dose of 30 μg/kg, diplopia and slight ptosis are sometimes evident but there are no other signs of muscular weakness.

During the initial phase of jitter increase there is sometimes a change in the MISI of up to about 1 ms. If this value increases the *second* potential shows blocking first; if the value decreases the *first* potential shows blocking.

After injection of Pancuronium bromide (Pavulon) similar effects are obtained (Stålberg and Hultman, unpublished). After the systemic injection of 1–2 mg (20 μg per kg body weight) the jitter increases rapidly in the next 30 seconds and in some recordings this proceeds to persistent blocking for about 10 minutes, and increased jitter may last as long as 40 minutes (Fig. 55).

When the jitter is increased owing to injection of such drugs, the interpotential intervals are distributed in a Gaussian fashion and are not dependent on the previous discharge interval. The mean innervation rate does, however, influence the jitter, which increases with a rising innervation rate. When there is partial blocking its degree increases at higher innervation rates. When the subject is asked to pause for a few seconds a few discharges may be obtained even when one of the potentials has previously shown total blocking (Fig. 56).

Within the limits 27–38°C the jitter increases with rising intramuscular temperature, more so when the initial value at the lower temperature is high.

The abnormal jitter produced by competitive blocking agents decreases after an injection of Edrophonium in the same way as it does in an abnormal potential pair in untreated myasthenia gravis.

The effect of a standard dose of curare on individual motor end-plates has been studied in some detail.[52] It has been shown that motor end-plates with an initially

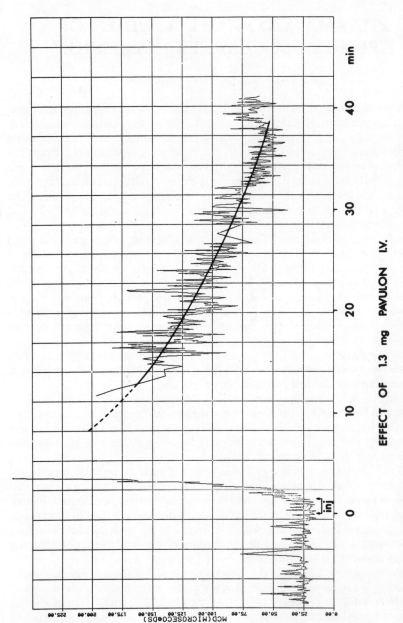

Fig. 55   Effect of 20 μg Pancuronium bromide (Pavulon) per kg body weight in normal subject. Ordinate: Jitter value (MCD). Abscissa: Time. Injection is made at time 0. Blocking occurs after 30 seconds and persists for about 12 minutes. The jitter is still abnormal 40 minutes thereafter. (Stålberg and Hultman, unpublished)

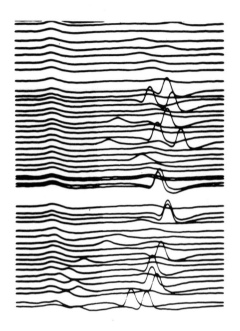

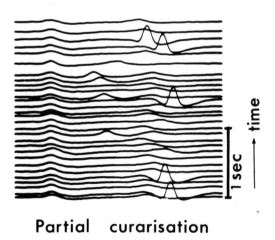

Partial   curarisation

Fig. 56   Disturbed neuromuscular transmission due to Pavulon. Note the transitional reappearance of the second potential after a short pause in voluntary activation.

small jitter are more resistant to curare than are those with an initially high normal jitter. Thus in a normal muscle the jitter value is correlated to the safety factor relative to curare. A motor end-plate with an initially increased jitter after pretreatment with curare shows increased responsiveness to a standard dose of curare. In other words a minimal dose of a competitive blocking agent will produce a larger than usual change in jitter values when the safety factor has been reduced by pretreatment with curare, and this fact can be made use of when drugs are being tested for their effect on neuromuscular transmission.

When testing drugs the action of which is not primarily upon neuromuscular transmission, uncomfortably high doses may have to be used. This can be avoided by prior regional curarization. A blood pressure cuff is placed around the upper arm and the pressure raised to 200 mm Hg. 0.5 mg d-Tubocurarine or a similar drug in 20 ml NaCl is injected into the dorsal vein of the arm. When the cuff is deflated after 5 to 10 minutes the subject does not usually experience any effects of the curare. When SFEMG recording is now started, most of the motor end-plates show increased jitter, which gradually normalises within 20 to 40 minutes. During this period a systemic injection of the drug to be tested can be given and even a very slight effect on neuromuscular transmission will be detected as an increase in the jitter.

DEPOLARIZING AGENTS

When injecting succinylcholine in small doses, say 2 to 6 mg intravenously, the subject experiences various degrees of fasciculation and sometimes slightly blurred vision. These effects usually disappear within 2 minutes. When SFEMG recordings are made with electrical stimulation the following events take place[58] (Fig. 57). After about 20 seconds there is a slight *latency decrease* of up to 0.1 ms. Then there is a more pronounced *latency increase*, 1.5 to 3.2 ms, after which the potential usually blocks. Depending on the dose, and the sensitivity of the motor end-plates under consideration, the blocking time may be up to 35 seconds. When the potential reappears, its latency remains increased for 5 to 20 seconds. During this time the jitter is also increased up to 120 μs, but gradually returns to normal values after 100 seconds. These results have been interpreted as follows:

The initial reduction in latency may be due to a slight depolarization, which shortens the time taken by the end-plate potential to reach the threshold. The subsequent increase in latency is probably due to a prolonged rise-time of the end-plate potential. The increase in latency and the abnormal jitter during the recovery phase seem to result from a reduced end-plate potential due to a desensitization to acetylcholine (in vitro experiments, Thesleff 1958).

When standard doses of succinylcholine are repeated at 15 minute intervals the effect is gradually diminished due to tachyphylaxis.

If a small dose of succinycholine is injected when recordings are being made from a motor end-plate pair with an initially increased jitter, the jitter decreases. This is true both when the initial increase in jitter is produced by pretreatment with small doses of curare, and in a muscle in which increased jitter is due to reinnervation. As suggested above, it is likely that this effect is due to a certain degree of membrane subdepolarization by succinycholine making it possible for a reduced and almost

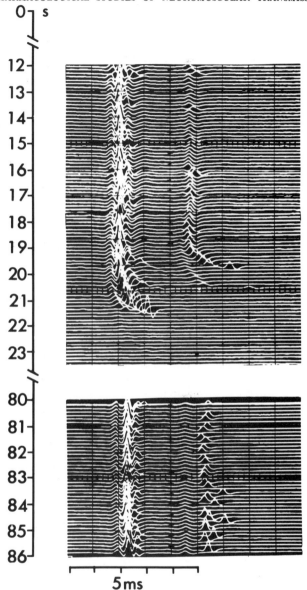

Fig. 57 Recording of action potentials from about six muscle fibres in the m. abductor digiti quinti on electrical stimulation of ulnar nerve (8 imp/s). The stimulus artefact, triggering the sweeps, is outside the figure. Five mg of succinylcholine was injected intravenously at 0. In the action potentials with the longest latency, an initial latency decrease is seen during the eighteenth second, followed by a latency increase and finally a block. The different action potentials disappear from 20 to 22s after injection. During recovery the jitter is still increased after 80–90s in the late action potential. MIPI is nearly normalized.

(From Stålberg, Thiele and Hilton-Brown, 1973)

insufficient end-plate potential to reach the trigger level more reliably and so facilitate transmission.

The time which elapses from the first change in latency to the point of blocking is usually only about one second, and it has consequently not been possible to measure the jitter value. This investigation therefore does not answer the question as to whether jitter studies may differentiate between partial anti-depolarizing and depolarizing block.

SFEMG FINDINGS IN DIFFERENT DISORDERS

DENERVATED MUSCLE

Fibrillation Potentials

In concentric needle EMG spontaneous activity in denervated muscle consists of fibrillation potentials and positive sharp waves. According to the prevailing view fibrillation potentials are due to the discharging of single denervated muscle fibres. Fibrillation potentials recorded in totally denervated muscle with an SFEMG electrode have the characteristics of the single fibre action potentials recorded in normal muscle[46, 77] (Fig. 58 A). Sometimes the negative or the positive peak of a fibrillation potential is a little rounder, but it usually satisfies the other criteria for single fibre action potentials (Fig. 58 B). Frequently the discharge rate is very uniform, sometimes with slowly and steadily increasing or decreasing frequency. When several different fibrillation potentials are being recorded, each usually fires at its own independent rate, but sometimes fibrillation potentials are seen to occur in pairs, closely time-locked to each other and with low jitter (Fig. 59). Such a finding can be interpreted in two ways: it may represent a split fibre, or the generation of the two action potentials by two different fibres, the second fibre being driven by the action potential of the first. Such ephaptic activation is conceivable in view of the decreased firing threshold of denervated muscle fibres. A finding which supports the latter possibility is illustrated in Fig. 60. Here two spontaneously occurring fibrillation potentials were recorded, each following its own rate. Potential No. 1 appeared with great regularity at 2.5 Hz, but potential No. 2 firing at 2 Hz was occasionally triggered by potential No. 1, sometimes twice in a row. This introduced irregularity into the otherwise very constant firing rate of potential No. 2, because the interval preceding the concomitant firing was shorter and the interval following the concomitant firing was longer, resembling an extrasystole and its compensatory pause in ECG. Apparently potential 1 provided an electrical stimulus which was strong enough to depolarise fibre 2 when it occurred in that fibre's supernormal period.

Bizarre High-frequency Discharges

This type of spontaneous activity, sometimes referred to as "pseudomyotonic bursts" is most commonly seen in muscles undergoing slowly progressive denervation. As is known from CNEMG it is usually provoked by movements of the needle electrode, consists of varying numbers of different spike components occurring at high, sometimes slightly diminishing, frequency and ceases abruptly.

In SFEMG recordings,[76] bizarre high-frequency discharges are often very complex potentials containing up to 10 or even more distinct single fibre action potentials separated by intervals ranging between less than 0.5 ms and as much as 100–200 ms. Usually in such a complex potential the mean interspike interval is

99

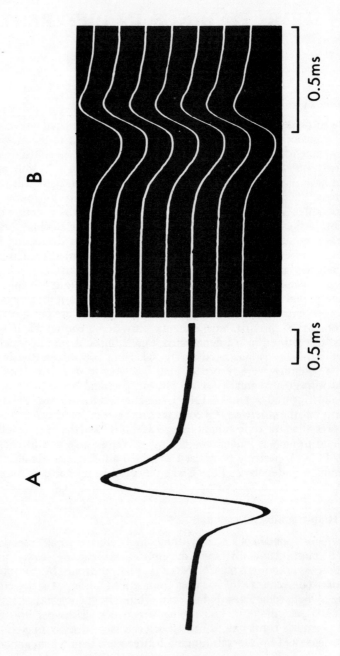

Fig. 58 Recordings from denervated muscle. A. A fibrillation potential, resembling a single fibre action potential (50 super-impositions). B. The occasional finding of a fibrillation potential with a slightly abnormal shape, in this case rounded positive peak.

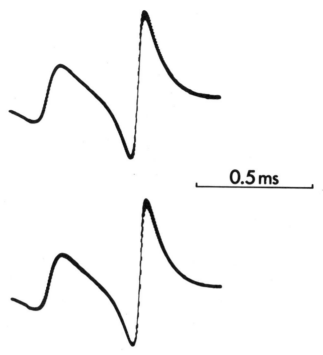

Fig. 59   A fibrillating pair of action potentials with jitter between 3 and 5 μs. 2
groups of 10 superimposed discharges.

considerably longer than in the normal muscle. With only few exceptions, the firing
order of the individual components remained constant, but the beginning and the
end of the complex (the cycle) were most often impossible to recognize before the
whole burst stopped. The firing rate of the complex as a whole ranged between about
5 and over 100 Hz.

In most instances the jitter between the different potentials in the complex
expressed as MCD was very small, 2–6 μs (Fig. 61), while there was frequently a
considerable slow trend, i.e. continuous lengthening or shortening of IPIs (Fig. 62).
On the other hand, variation of successive interdischarge intervals was frequently
also very small. Here slow trends were more obvious.

One or several action potentials of the whole group might transiently show
increased jitter with or without blocking, particularly immediately before
disappearing from the complex, or just after reappearing. When several action
potentials behaved in this way, the large jitter and blocking were usually concomitant.
MCD of the IDIs increased considerably just before the whole burst stopped.

It is assumed that the burst is initiated by one fibre in the complex which serves as a
pacemaker for one or several other fibres; it excites them ephaptically by its own

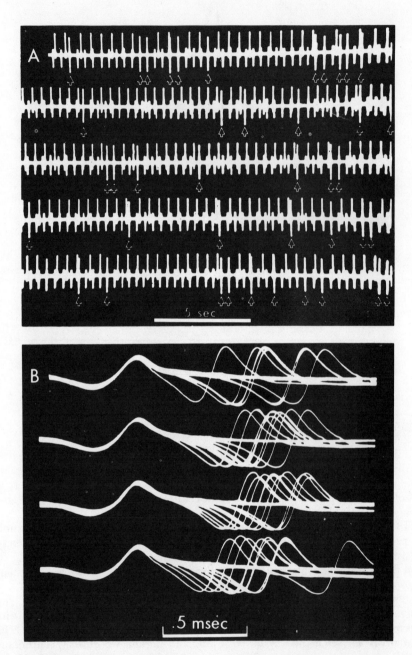

Fig. 60 Two fibrillation potentials, sometimes locked (arrows in A). This phenomenon is shown in more detail in B. (From Trontelj, Stålberg and Janko, 1975)

A   B

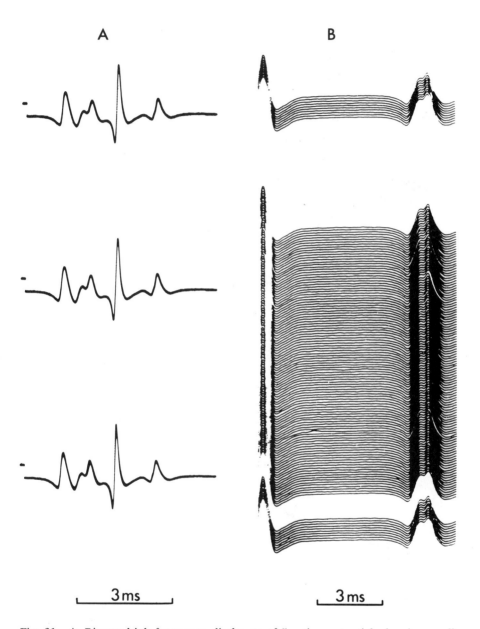

3 ms   3 ms

Fig. 61 A. Bizarre high-frequency discharge of 5 action potentials showing small
jitter on superimposed recordings (10x). B. Another multispike recording
with small jitter with two abrupt intermissions during otherwise regular
high frequency (80 c/s) discharges.

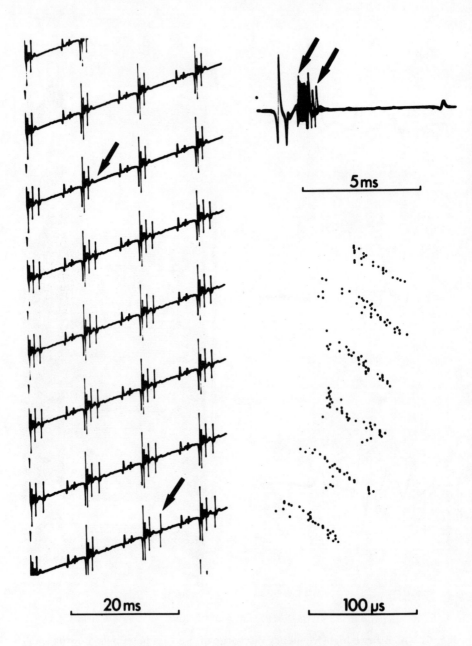

Fig. 62 Action potentials and sequential histogram of a spontaneous high-frequency discharge. Note progressive lengthening of the IPI until a block occurs, followed by a repeated sequence. (Time downwards in histogram)

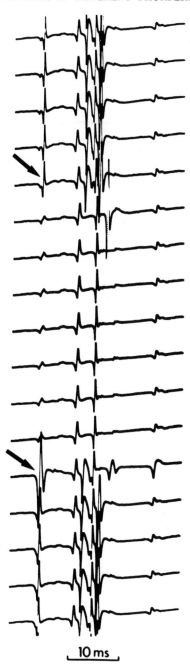

Fig. 63 Temporary blocking (between arrows) of a group of fibres in a bizarre high frequency discharge. This group is presumably driven by a secondary pacemaker fibre. Sweep moved upwards.

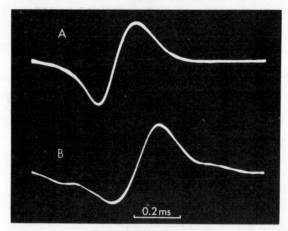

Fig. 64   A. Superimposition of 50 discharges of a fibrillation potential.
B. The same muscle fibre driven by an electrical stimulus applied close to
the recording electrode. Now also some other fibres are activated which
results in slight change of the action potential shape.

action potential. In the next cycle the principal pacemaker fibre is probably excited in turn by one of the later fibres' action potential in the first cycle (co-principal pacemaker), and the whole cycle is repeated at high frequency. This results in cumulative decreased excitability leading first to intermittent and later to permanent blocking of individual fibres or sometimes groups of fibres, which are apparently activated by secondary pacemakers (Fig. 63). Sometimes all fibres block intermittently together, so that one complete cycle out of two or three is missing. In that case the principal pacemaker fibre is perhaps not detected by the recording electrode. The whole burst stops abruptly when either the principal or the co-principal pacemaker fibre becomes sufficiently subnormal to block.

In contrast to most fibrillation potentials, the single fibre action potentials in bizarre high-frequency discharges are frequently of rather high amplitude, which indicates absence of atrophy or even suggests work hypertrophy, developed prior to denervation to compensate for the loss of previously denervated motor units, and perhaps maintained by the continued activity after denervation. If the hypothesis of ephaptic activation is correct, then large action potentials with their stronger electrical field more easily depolarize adjacent fibres. The rather long MISI is explained by scattering of the low threshold sites at which the different muscle fibres become depolarized. This scattering is conceivably wider than that of the motor end-plates in the normal muscle.

At present, explanations of the phenomenon of bizarre high-frequency discharges alternative to the ephaptic activation of muscle fibres are difficult to conceive. One possibility would be spontaneous activity in excessively split muscle fibres.

Electrical Stimulation of Denervated Muscle Fibres

When a spontaneously firing fibrillation potential is detected with a single fibre EMG electrode it is often possible to place a monopolar stimulating electrode a few millimetres or centimetres further along the course of the muscle fibre in such a position that now the same fibrillation potential is driven by the electrical stimuli[78] (Fig. 64). The depolarisation of denervated muscle fibres by electrical stimulus is quite easily achieved when the duration of the electrical pulses is 10 ms or longer. It is possible to use much shorter pulses, down to 50 μs or less, but then the position of the stimulating electrode becomes critical.

When the stimulus strength is near threshold, the latency variation in the responses is extremely large, sometimes in the range of several thousand μs, but when the stimulus is well above threshold the jitter becomes small, less than 2–5 μs (Fig. 65). With continuously increasing stimulus strength new potentials usually enter; their jitter is large at first but with further increase of stimulus strength it becomes small. The decrease in jitter is associated with a shortening of latency. Conversely, lengthening of latencies and increase in jitter occurs on decreasing the stimulus strength. Nearly always this change in latency is more or less smooth, but sometimes it occurs in steps. The continuous decrease of the jitter and the shortening of the latency when raising the stimulus strength are similar to those occurring in the stimulated nerve fibre, but usually more pronounced (page 27).

The stepwise latency change on increasing or decreasing stimulus strength can be explained in the following way. Some denervated fibres are not uniformly susceptible to electrical stimulation along their entire course but have sites of significantly lower threshold (Thesleff, 1977). When on increasing the stimulus strength the electrical field spreads out, it is too weak to start an action potential between two low threshold sites, but when it is increased a little more, the starting point of the action potential jumps from the nearer site to the more distant site with a resulting stepwise shortening of the latency. Another possibility would be stimulation of two branches of split fibre with different propagation velocities. In some cases the stepwise shortening of the latency was clearly associated with the appearance of another fibre in the response, and the lengthening of the latency with the disappearance of that fibre (Fig. 66). In such cases the fibre's action potential may have discharged the fibre with the bimodal latency phenomenon at one of the low threshold sites which has already been subdepolarised by the stimulus. This explanation would imply that the action potential of a muscle fibre can significantly influence the threshold of another muscle fibre or even depolarise it by the mechanisms of ephaptic transmission, as suggested by the spontaneous occurrence of pairs of fibrillation potentials and the intermittently time-locked fibrillation potentials as well as by the bizarre high-frequency discharges described above.

Again an alternative possibility is recording from one branch of a split muscle fibre, activated once directly and once through the other branch, rather as in the case of the axon reflex. This, however, would not explain the association of the phenomenon with appearance and disappearance of another fibre's responses.

Some denervated fibres could follow stimulation with one response to each stimulus at rates as high as 200/s, sometimes for long periods. Usually they showed rapid exhaustion, evident as progressively increasing latency and increasing rise time of the action potential (Fig. 67).

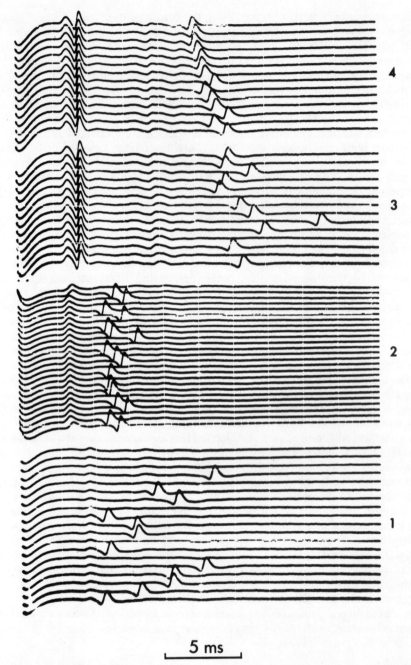

5 ms

Fig. 65   Electrical stimulation in denervated muscle at increasing stimulus strengths
(1–4) showing large jitter at threshold and low jitter a suprathreshold
stimulus, as well as shortening of the latencies.

REINNERVATION

Reinnervation of a denervated muscle can take place in two ways. One is by the outgrowth of new motor axons, which is possible when, after a traumatic lesion, the continuity of the nerve fascicles has been preserved or re-established. In this case, the regenerating axons must traverse new and at times tortuous pathways and may reach the denervated muscle at widely separated times. After the arriving axon has innervated a muscle fibre, it develops branches that supply a group of adjacent denervated muscle fibres, and subsequently entering axons act in a similar manner. In this way compact motor units are formed (Romanul and van der Meulen, 1967). Kugelberg, Edström and Abruzzese (1970) have shown that in this type of reinnervation the average motor unit may contain approximately the same number of muscle fibres as in the normal muscle, in which case most motor axons have taken part in reinnervation.

The second type of reinnervation occurs after partial denervation. This is followed by mainly subterminal collateral sprouting of nerve twigs from neighbouring healthy motor axons (Hoffman, 1950; Edds, 1950). The stimulus to collateral sprouting is not obvious, but it has been suggested that it may be due to a loss of an inhibitory factor provided via centripetal axonal transport from the normal muscle.

Mitotic activity in the nerve stumps reaches a maximum about 3 weeks after nerve section (Abercrombie and Johnson, 1942, 1946). If the residual and degenerating nerve fibres lie near to each other, cell proliferation might provide a stimulus for collateral sprouting (Edds, 1950). Van Harreveld (1945) suggested that the reinnervation is due to a general stimulus by agents liberated from the denervated muscle.

Coërs and Woolf (1959) observed that one single terminal nerve fibre can supply as many as 19 end-plates in peripheral neuropathy, as opposed to one or two in normal muscle. Clusters of reinnervated muscle fibres appear in proximity to the muscle fibres of surviving motor units from which the collateral sprouting has taken place, so that the number of muscle fibres belonging to each motor unit may increase considerably in the process of reinnervation (Wohlfart, 1958). They appear as scattered groups of fibres showing in histochemical preparations as fibre type grouping (Karpati and Engel, 1968; Morris, 1969), and not as the compact clusters seen after outgrowth of a new motor axon. The muscle fibres of a normal motor unit are distributed in a number of fascicles and are intermingled with muscle fibres of other motor units. When collateral reinnervation has taken place the boundaries of the increased motor units coincide to a large extent with the boundaries of fascicles, suggesting that the healthy motor unit does not supply collaterals to denervated muscle fibres outside the fascicles in which it was originally represented, probably because collateral sprouting is hindered by the intramuscular connective tissue (Kugelberg, Edström and Abruzzese, 1970). This, clearly, does not apply when a lesion high up the nerve trunk leads to collateral axonal sprouting (Gilliatt, 1966) or to the faulty re-innervation of facial muscles which may follow Bell's palsy.

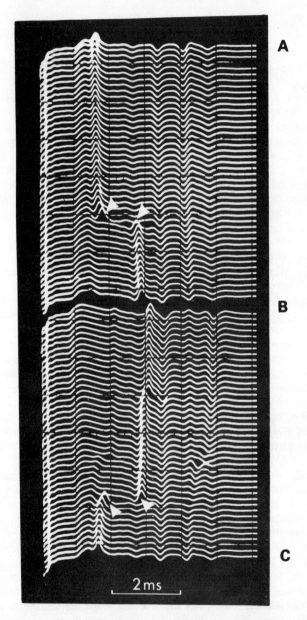

Fig. 66   (Above and top on facing page) Responses of denervated muscle fibres to electrical stimulation (2 Hz, 50 μs). The stimulus was decreasing in very small steps from A to B and increasing again from B to C. Notice stepwise latency change of one of the fibres (full arrows), associated with disappearance and reappearance of another fibre (empty arrows in the recording at the head of the facing page).

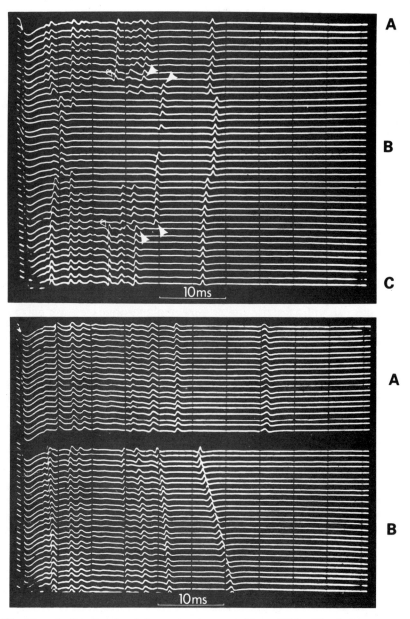

Fig. 67 Electrically stimulated denervated muscle fibres (5 Hz, 50 μs). A: responses following about 20 seconds of continuous stimulation, which resulted in increasing subnormality, seen in increased latency and action potential duration. B: a short resting period is followed by a partial and short latency recovery. Fibres No. 2, 3, and 7 show a little shorter latency in the second response after rest, indicating slightly supernormal VRF.

MULTI-ELECTRODE STUDIES OF THE MOTOR UNIT IN
MOTOR NEURONE DISEASE AND POLYNEUROPATHIES

SFEMG multi-electrode investigations using the technique described (page 87) have been made with the purpose of mapping muscle fibre distribution within the reinnervated human motor unit.[40] Glycogen depletion studies are obviously impracticable, and the histochemical demonstration of fibre type grouping does not tell us of the relation between different parts of the motor unit. In patients with motor neurone disease 27 motor unit recordings in the EDC muscle (Fig. 68) were made. There was an increased average fibre density over the reference electrode of 2.0–5.0 as compared to the normal mean of 1.4 (SD 0.2). There were 4 or more fibres over the reference electrode in 15 (56%) of the recordings, whereas the maximum number in the normal study was 3 fibres. The average number of fibres in the corridors was 7.8–24.8 for the individual patients (normal mean 3.9, SD 0.8). There were 7 corridors (26%) with 10 or more fibres; in the normals the maximum was 9 fibres. In 1 motor unit corridor there were 3 fibres recorded and the next lowest had 4 fibres. There were no corridors in which only the reference electrode was active, though this was found in 24% of the corridors in normals.

In some corridors, especially in patients with marked weakness and denervation, there were groups of fibres over many adjacent electrodes. Occasionally groups of action potentials with a fast rise time and low amplitude were seen over only a single electrode. The study was made in biceps brachii muscle in only one patient (Fig. 68 B). There was moderate weakness and denervation of this muscle. An increased number of fibres were recorded on average over the reference electrode (3.7) and within the corridors (13.7).

The study was also performed in seven patients with polyneuropathy (two of unknown aetiology, one alcoholic, one diabetic and three with Charcot-Marie-Tooth disease). In EDC 37 motor unit corridors were recorded (Fig. 69 A). The average fibre density over the reference electrode was 2.8–8.8 (normal mean 1.5, SD 0.2) and the average number of fibres in the corridors was 7.2–38.7 (normal mean 3.9, SD 0.8). Nine motor units (24%) had 4 or more fibres over the reference electrode and 19 motor units (51%) had 10 or more fibres in an individual corridor. The fibre density and numbers of fibres in the corridor were highest in the patients with Charcot-Marie-Tooth disease. A number of corridors showed groups of two or more fibres over single electrodes. There were several corridors with groups of fibres over adjacent electrodes and in one corridor in a patient with chronic polyneuropathy (I.B. in Fig. 69) 65 fibres over the central electrodes (2 mm) were recorded. In the biceps brachii (Fig. 69 B) the average fibre density was increased to 1.7–3.2 (normal mean 1.3, SD 0.2) as was the average number of fibres in the corridors, 6.3–8.5 (normal mean 3.7, SD 1.3). Although there were only 3 of 13 motor units (23%) showing one or the other definite criterion of abnormality (more than 9 fibres in the corridor or more than 3 fibres over an electrode) the average value for the parameters was abnormal in each patient, since some of the motor units had values near the upper normal limit.

In both motor neurone disease and polyneuropathy there tended to be more fibres in the corridor when there were more fibres recorded over the reference electrode (Table 8).

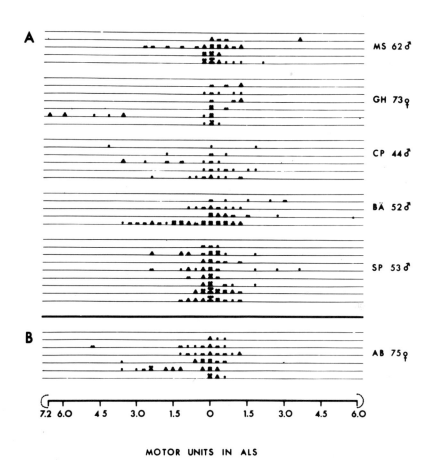

MOTOR UNITS IN ALS

Fig. 68 Motor unit corridors in motor neurone disease recorded from EDC (A) and biceps brachii muscles (B). Each dot represents a different single muscle fibre action potential. The initial reference electrode (6) is at distance 0. There is prominent grouping in some of the corridors, e.g. in the 8th corridor in patient SP, where there are 7 fibres over the reference electrode and 7 additional over the adjacent electrodes, 300 μm to either side. (From Schwartz, Stålberg, Schiller and Thiele, 1976)

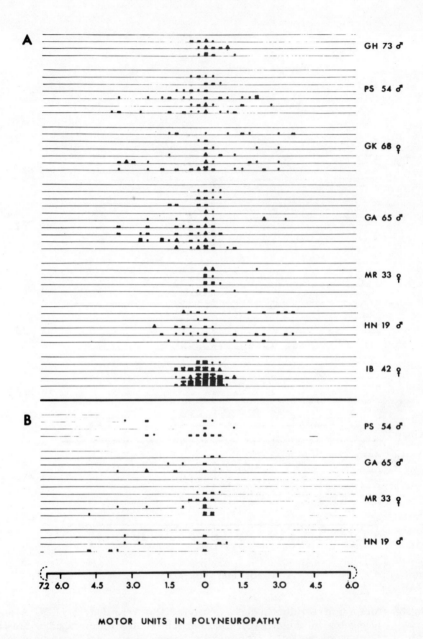

MOTOR UNITS IN POLYNEUROPATHY

Fig. 69   Motor unit corridors in polyneuropathy from EDC (A) and biceps brachii muscles (B). Grouping is particularly prominent in recordings from patient IB with chronic polyneuropathy.
(From Schwartz, Stålberg, Schiller and Thiele, 1976)

No. of fibres over reference electrode	No. of additional fibres in the corridor					
	normal		MND		PN	
	mean	n	mean	n	mean	n
EDC						
1	2.1	(36)	2.0	(1)	10.0	(3)
2	2.9	(12)	5.1	(8)	6.0	(1)
3	3.4	(5)	7.7	(3)	7.9	(12)
4			13.1	(7)	3.3	(3)
5			5.8	(4)	15.0	(2)
6			—		6.0	(1)
7			16.7	(3)	—	
8			—		29	(1)
9					31	(1)
12					56	(1)
Biceps brachii						
1	1.4	(36)	—		3.0	(1)
2	3.5	(11)			3.8	(8)
3	5.0	(11)	9.0	(3)	8.5	(2)
4			17.5	(2)	4.0	(2)
5			4.0	(1)		

Table 8. Distribution of muscle fibres along the multielectrode corridor in motoneurone disease (MND) and polyneuropathies (PN) in comparison to normal. No. in brackets denotes number of corridors studied.

"Motor Unit Territory"

The maximal distance between muscle fibres in a single corridor in motor neurone disease was 7 mm in EDC (6 mm in normals) and 5.5 mm in the biceps brachii muscle (6–7 mm in normals). In polyneuropathy it was 7 mm in EDC and 5 mm in the biceps brachii muscles. For reasons already given (page 91), this method is not suitable for determining the actual boundaries of the motor unit territory. Nevertheless the increased fibre density in polyneuropathies to some extent compensates for the methodological drawbacks, and the values obtained for the maximal distance between muscle fibres in the recording corridor are probably quite close to the actual diameter of the motor unit territory in the corresponding plane.

Comments on the Multi-electrode Findings

The most common abnormal finding in this study was the increased number of double and triple action potentials within the corridors. The increased fibre density values found in patients with anterior horn cell disease[54] and alcoholic polyneuropathy[64] reflect these changes. In the clinically more affected muscles even larger groups of fibres were recorded. The most pronounced grouping was found in one of the patients with Charcot-Marie-Tooth disease (cf. a CNEMG study by Hayward and Willison, 1977). In the study of the normal motor unit[53] it was shown that when there were more fibres over the reference electrode there was a tendency for more fibres to be recorded in the corridor. In the reinnervated motor units the same tendency was present but grouping was now evident.

The size of the motor unit territory was not given particular attention in this investigation. The recording corridor is narrow, and muscle fibres near the boundary of the motor unit, which should be recorded for territory measurements, are easily missed. In principle, underestimation of territorial extent should not wholly invalidate conclusions as to the size of the motor unit drawn from the maximal distances between responses along the corridors on many insertions, since in cases of collateral sprouting the chance of recording muscle fibres at the periphery of the motor unit increases. In the present investigation the longest distances between the responses obtained were not greater than in normal subjects, even though fibre density was increased, so that no indication of increased size of the motor unit territory was obtained in these patients. This finding is in agreement with those of Kugelberg, Edström and Abruzzese (1970) in rats, where a particular motor unit showed collateral sprouting only within those fascicles where it was originally represented.

The physiological changes accompanying reinnervation seem to occur before histochemical changes are evident in the muscle fibre. Studies with experimental reinnervation in the cat (Hakelius, Nyström and Stålberg, 1975) and rat (Warszawski, Telerman-Toppet, Durdu, Graff and Coërs, 1975) have demonstrated that function and normal twitch characteristics returned to reinnervated muscle fibres as early as two weeks before differentiation of fibre types could be made with ATP-ase reaction.

In summary, the distribution of fibres in the reinnervated motor unit in this study is in agreement with the glycogen depletion studies following reinnervation in the rat (Kugelberg, Edström and Abruzzese, 1970). Our results show that the reinnervated motor unit in man is similar to that demonstrated in the experimental animal and is in accord with the interpretation put on histochemical findings in man. The multi-electrode study has demonstrated that a correlation exists between the number of fibres in individual corridors and the number of fibres recorded over individual electrode surfaces which applies both to the normal and to pathological muscle. This means that for practical purposes fibre density studies with a single electrode surface (see page 64) can give information about the abnormal distribution of muscle fibres in the motor unit as satisfactory as can be obtained in the more complicated multi-electrode investigation.

SINGLE-SURFACE SFEMG RECORDINGS IN REINNERVATION
(MUSCLE TRANSPLANTS)

To study the process of reinnervation SFEMG recordings have been made in muscle transplants in neurologically healthy patients[25] and animals (Hakelius, Nyström and Stålberg, 1976) when the time at which reinnervation begins can be relatively well defined. One month after muscle transplantation the first action potentials are recorded from voluntarily activated muscle fibres with increased jitter and frequent blocking. The degree of blocking decreases and is seen only rarely after six months. The jitter decreases at the same time. The fibre density increases during the first six months, particularly the first three. The blocking and increased jitter indicate uncertain transmission in the immature nerve twigs and motor end-plates. The increase in fibre density is taken as an effect of increasing sprouting with adoption of new muscle fibres.

These two parameters can therefore be used to follow the stage and extent of reinnervation (Fig. 70). Recordings with blocking and increased jitter suggest that reinnervation has probably taken place during the previous three months. Recordings with increased fibre density and stable reinnervation complexes indicate that little or no reinnervation has taken place during the previous six months. It should be noted that these conclusions are drawn from the investigation of healthy nerve and muscle fibres. Whether reinnervation in nerve and muscle disorders proceeds at the same rate and to the same stage of functional maturity is not yet known.

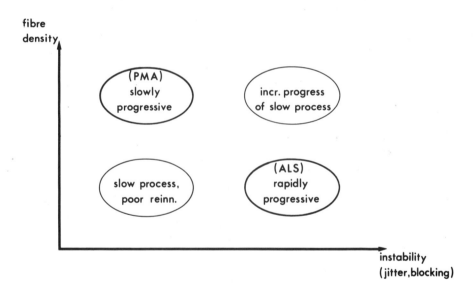

Fig. 70 Schematic illustration of the SFEMG findings in processes with collateral sprouting. Increase in fibre density (a correlate to morphology) indicates the degree of reinnervation, most pronounced in slow processes allowing time for axonal sprouting and reinnervation. Large jitter and blocking of individual spike components (a functional parameter) indicates recently reinnervated muscle fibres. There is a pronounced instability during the first 3 months of reinnervation, a finding typical of rapidly progressive disorder. Intermediate forms are also possible.
(From Stålberg, 1976)

ANTERIOR HORN CELL DISORDERS

In anterior horn cell disorders[54] the *fibre density* is increased, particularly in the more slowly advancing types such as spinal muscular atrophy and syringomyelia, in which there is time for the outgrowth of a rich network of collateral sprouts resulting in large motor units. In the more rapid processes the reinnervating motor unit may die before effective sprouting has developed, or the surviving motor neurones may be sick and incapable of supporting new sprouts. The fibre density values obtained in a small series of patients were: in amyotrophic lateral sclerosis 3.3, in spinal muscular atrophy 6.2, in Kugelberg-Welander disease 4.4, and in syringomyelia 4.7. *Increased jitter and blocking* are commonly seen in the rapidly progressive disorders such as amyotrophic lateral sclerosis, probably indicating continuous denervation and reinnervation with little time for forming mature sprouts and motor end-plates. Moreover in some disorders the motor neurones may never be capable of doing that, even after long survival. The duration of complex action potentials is always prolonged but the MISI is not greatly increased, particularly in the rapid processes. Most of the single fibre components are found early in the complex where they may be superimposed on one another to such a degree as to make it impossible to estimate their number. In the slowly progressive forms one or a few late components (referred to by some authors as "satellite" or "parasitic" potentials), often of low amplitude, are found in many complex potentials, increasing the MISI value. The propagation velocity in the later components is progressively lower for components with increasing delay after the initial part of the complex. This indicates that at least one reason for the long delay of the late components is that they derive from small muscle fibres with low propagation velocity.

The dual finding of increased fibre density and unstable complex configuration suggests a rapidly progressive process of active reinnervation, as in amyotrophic lateral sclerosis (Fig. 71 A). A combination of very much increased fibre density and stable complexes, particularly stable in the initial part, indicates a slowly progressive disorder or a burned-out process with marked long-standing reinnervation (Fig. 71 B).

The combination of high fibre density and unstable impulse conduction with complexes of long duration may occur in the case of exacerbation of a chronic neurogenic process (Fig. 71 C).

Another such example is that of a patient with long-standing weakness after poliomyelitis beginning to deteriorate; in this case the finding described may be due to premature dying of the motoneurones with attempts to compensate by further reinnervation, although quantitatively insufficient. We cannot exclude in these cases the possibility that the increased jitter and blocking are due to a degenerative process within the motor unit studied.

In any single case with one of the above diagnoses the SFEMG results may overlap those of another group. Nevertheless the findings may be used to characterise the functional status of the motor unit, the extent and effectiveness of reinnervation, and the degree of stability of neuromuscular function. This information may contribute to diagnostic precision and to the assessment of prognosis.

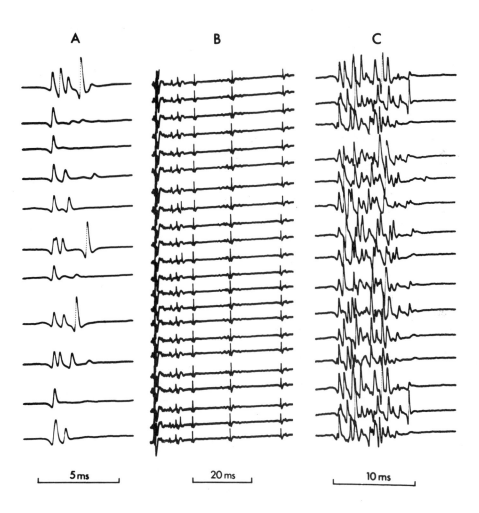

Fig. 71   A. Recording from a patient with amyotrophic lateral sclerosis. Five spike components forming a very unstable complex with intermittent blocking of at least four components. B. Stable multiple potential in a patient with long-standing nonprogressive neurogenic disorder. C. Unstable complex potential in a patient with long-standing deteriorating poliomyelitis.

MYASTHENIA GRAVIS

The concept of an auto-immune pathogenesis of myasthenia gravis is now generally accepted (Heilbronn, Mallson and Stålberg, 1974; Heilbronn and Stålberg, 1978).

Clinical and neurophysiological tests for the diagnosis of myasthenia gravis are based on the occurrence of neuromuscular blocking, defined as failure of transmission at a proportion of individual motor end-plates. By means of SFEMG neuromuscular disturbances can be detected as increased jitter (Fig. 72) before impulse blocking occurs and thus before symptoms are present.[18,46,48,61] The recording can be made during voluntary activity or electrical stimulation.[26]

Voluntary Activity

Twenty potential pairs is a convenient number to investigate in each muscle. Disturbed neuromuscular transmission can be detected with fewer recordings, but to quantitate the abnormality this number of recordings should be made. In the more severely affected patient this can be difficult. The typical findings in a patient with myasthenia include usually within any one muscle:[48,61] 1. motor end-plates with normal jitter values, 2. jitter values above the normal range but without impulse blocking, and 3. recordings with increased jitter and intermittent impulse blocking which usually first appears with a jitter around 100 μs (Fig. 73). Here the range between the maximal and minimal interpotential interval in one potential pair at 50 discharges might be as large as 4000 μs (Fig. 74).

The study in each muscle is considered to have given a normal result if all, or all but one, of twenty recorded potential pairs have jitter values below that given as the upper normal limit (Table 4). Increased jitter, even with blocking, may occasionally be found in one out of twenty recordings in normal subjects. If jitter is normal in all fibre pairs but fewer than twenty have been recorded the study cannot be considered adequate. Even when the disease is very mild or confined to other muscles, usually more than 30% of potential pairs are abnormal in EDC. If the jitter is normal in a clinically weak muscle the diagnosis of myasthenia can be excluded. In cases of purely ocular myasthenia gravis a facial muscle such as frontalis may have to be sampled, since recordings in EDC may not show conclusive abnormality; this was the case in 2 out of 13 of our patients,[61] and in 3 out of 10 reported by Sanders, Howard and Johns (1978). So far we have investigated no patients with purely ocular myasthenia in whom jitter has been entirely normal in facial muscles. One patient with isolated swallowing difficulty, where the diagnosis of myasthenia was suggested by antibody titre against cholinergic receptors, showed normal jitter values in the EDC and frontalis muscles, but a few abnormal values in an incomplete study of masseter and temporalis muscles.

Concerning the possibility of a false positive diagnosis it must be made abundantly clear that increased jitter usually indicates disturbed neuro-muscular transmission but not exclusively the diagnosis of myasthenia gravis. Other causes will be discussed in the following chapters.

While the SFEMG investigation seeks to establish the proportion of normal, abnormally jittering and blocking pairs, the figure for the average jitter value is not entirely without interest. Thus, a small general influence on neuromuscular transmission exerted, for example, by a drug, may be seen as a slight but significant increase in the mean jitter value, though not beyond the upper limit for the normal population in the individual recordings.

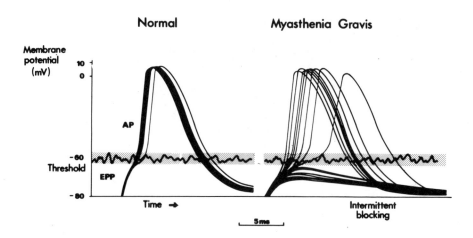

Fig. 72   Schematic drawing explaining the phenomenon of neuromuscular jitter, based on an intracellular recording from human intercostal muscle fibre (Elmqvist, Hofmann, Kugelberg and Quastel, 1964). In the normal muscle fibre, the changes in neuromuscular transmission time are due to the fluctuation of the threshold value of membrane potential at which the muscle fibre becomes depolarized when this value is reached by the end-plate potential (EPP). In myasthenic muscle fibre, the end-plate potentials are less steep and their amplitude is variable. Some of them fail to reach the triggering threshold and no action potential (AP) is generated (intermittent transmission blocking). (From Stålberg, Trontelj and Schwartz, 1976)

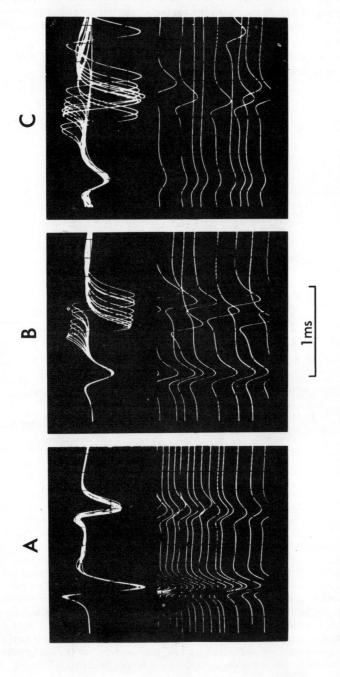

1ms

Fig. 73 SFEMG jitter recordings from extensor digitorum communis muscle of a patient with myasthenia gravis. The oscilloscope sweep is triggered by the first action potential and the interval variability between the single fibre potentials (the neuromuscular jitter) is seen as a variable position of the second potential. In the upper row 10 action potentials are superimposed. In the lower row the oscilloscope sweep is moved downwards. In (A) normal jitter, in (B) increased jitter but no impulse blockings and in (C) increased jitter and occasional blockings. (From Stålberg, Trontelj and Schwartz, 1976)

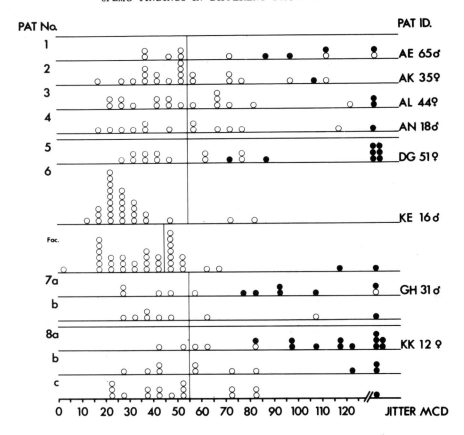

Fig. 74   Jitter recordings from the extensor digitorum communis muscle (EDC)
(and in addition from the facial muscle in one case) in eight patients with
myasthenia gravis. Each horizontal line is one investigation and each dot is
the jitter in one potential pair calculated from more than 200 discharges.
Filled circles indicate recordings with partial blocking. The vertical line is
the upper normal limit of the jitter value. Patients 1–4 have generalized
symptoms, 1 and 2 untreated, 3 and 4 on anticholinesterase therapy. Note
the range of jitter values from normal to very abnormal including
blockings. Patients 5, 6 and 7 have only ocular symptoms. Patient 6 is the
one in our material with the fewest abnormal recordings in EDC. In his
frontalis muscle (Fac.) a larger proportion of abnormal potential pairs was
found. Patients 7 and 8 are included to show the effect of treatment: 7a and
8a, untreated; 7b and 8b, on anticholinesterase therapy 1–2 months after
thymectomy with clinical improvement and only slight fatiguability; 8c on
medical treatment 2 years later but without symptoms or signs of
fatiguability. Note the reduction in numbers of recordings with blocking
after therapy. Abnormal jitter values are however still obtained.
(From Stålberg, Trontelj and Schwartz, 1976)

In a study of 70 patients with myasthenia gravis, Sanders, Howard and Johns (1978) reported a good correlation between SFEMG abnormalities and the clinical classification of myasthenia when the recordings were made from the extensor digitorum communis muscle, confirming that the porportion of motor end-plates with abnormal transmission is higher in patients with greater clinical weakness. Positive correlation is found between clinical fatiguability and number of potential pairs showing blocking both when the patients are untreated, and when they are treated with cholinesterase inhibitors or steroids.

In serial studies also, the severity of the SFEMG abnormalities often showed good correlation with changes in clinical weakness, for example after corticosteroid treatment, especially when intervals between successive studies were longer than one month (D.B. Sanders, personal communication).

The two-needle technique was employed to study more than two muscle fibres belonging to the same motor unit[61] (page 31). One electrode was kept in a constant position throughout the whole investigation of that motor unit and the recorded action potential triggered the oscilloscope sweep. Another electrode was moved in the muscle until it was recording an action potential time-locked to the triggering one, i.e. the electrodes were recording action potentials from muscle fibres of the same motor unit.

The jitter was measured between the triggering potential of the constant electrode and the potentials obtained with the second electrode. Up to seven motor end-plates were studied within the same motor unit. In muscles in which a range of normal and abnormal jitter values had been obtained in ordinary one-needle recordings, the same range of jitter values was seen within a single motor unit (Fig. 75). No tendency to homogeneous involvement or to sparing of the motor unit as a whole could be detected.

An initially abnormal jitter may increase during continuous activity, particularly at increasing innervation rates. When the innervation rate again decreases, the jitter and degree of blocking also fall. When one of the potentials shows a high degree of blocking at a high innervation rate it is more likely to reappear when the preceding interdischarge interval is long (Fig. 76). An initially normal jitter does not usually change during activity. Sometimes a decrease in jitter and blocking is seen at increasing innervation rate, and occasionally recruitment of activity from other muscle fibres belonging to the motor unit under study.

After the injection of Edrophonium (Tensilon) the normal jitter remains unchanged. In an abnormal potential pair the blockings disappear and the jitter tends to return towards the normal value without quite achieving it[68] (Fig. 77). Occasionally the reverse Edrophonium effect, namely increased jitter and more frequent blocking, can be observed in a muscle with an otherwise positive response to the drug. This is especially true when the patient is on anticholinesterase treatment.

Exceptionally, all SFEMG parameters become normal during clinical remission, either spontaneous or following thymectomy or corticosteroid therapy (Sanders, Howard and Johns, 1978; Stålberg and Trontelj, unpublished). During improvement with anticholinesterase therapy there is no complete normalisation of values. It follows that it is not necessary to have the patient off anticholinesterase medication to detect the myasthenic disturbance. It is our experience that most patients who on clinical grounds are in complete remission after treatment still show a certain proportion of potential pairs with increased jitter but almost no blocking.

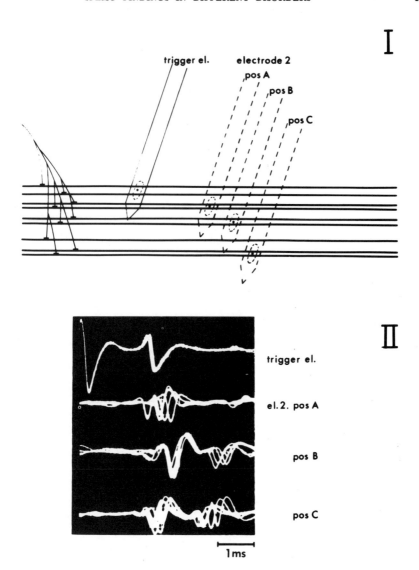

Fig. 75   Recordings from 7 muscle fibres in frontalis muscle from a patient with
myasthenia gravis. It shows the two-needle recording technique. Trigger
electrode kept in constant position close to two muscle fibres in the motor
unit triggering the oscilloscope sweep (II, trigger el.). Electrode 2 is moved
to three different positions where activity from muscle fibres belonging to
the triggering motor unit is obtained (II). Three of the motor end-plates
(the two obtained with a triggering electrode and the first in position B)
have a normal jitter, three have an increased jitter without blocking (A, B,
C) and one has increased jitter with blocking (the last in position C).
(From Stålberg, Trontelj and Schwartz, 1976)

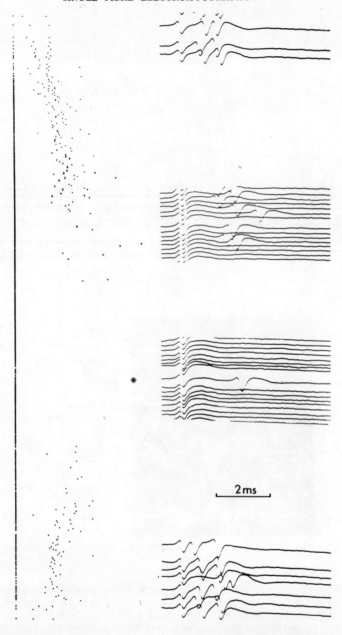

Fig. 76 SFEMG recording in a patient with myasthenia gravis at different voluntary innervation rates. The three spike components are represented as dots. Time downwards. Note the increasing MIPI and degree of blocking during continuous high innervation rate and recovery when the rate is lowered again. During the period of total block, a short pause is enough to relieve blocking of one of the spikes for one discharge (asterisk).

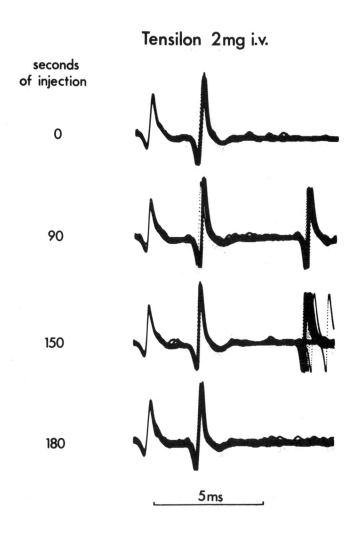

Fig. 77   Effect of an intravenous injection of 2mg Tensilon in a myasthenic patient.
A fibre previously fatigued to total block reappears with only moderately
increased jitter at 90s after injection. At 150s the jitter increases and there is
intermittent blocking. At 2 min. after injection the fibre is in complete block
again.

An anticholinesterase given to a healthy subject in similar doses as those used in treatment of myasthenia does not produce any significant effect on the jitter. We do not believe in the possibility of false positive findings, i.e. abnormal jitter in healthy subjects receiving anticholinesterase medication. This opinion is based on experience with a patient who had been on anticholinesterase drugs for years due to erroneous diagnosis of myasthenia gravis but still had normal SFEMG. Moreover, a group of pesticide workers tested before and after exposure to an organophosphorous compound giving rise to a slight but significant change in esterase activity had jitter values unchanged.[51] With heavy doses producing intoxication, however, it is reasonable to expect increased jitter.

In about 25% of the patients the fibre density was slightly but significantly increased above normal values (Fig. 78). In very weak muscle the fibre density may be underestimated, owing to permanent block of a proportion of muscle fibres. The finding of increased fibre density may reflect reinnervation after denervation due to the myasthenic process or, more likely, is an effect of anticholinesterase treatment. Abnormal motor end-plates are seen histologically (Coërs and Woolf, 1959) and pronounced changes have been demonstrated in electron-microscopic studies both in human (Engel, 1977) and in experimentally induced myasthenia (Heilbronn, Mattson, Thornell, Sjöström, Stålberg, Hilton-Brown and Elmqvist, 1976; Engel, Tsujihata, Sakakibara, Lindstrom and Lambert, 1977). Morphological and physiological (Engel, Lambert and Santa, 1973; Roberts and Thesleff, 1969) changes of motor end-plates have been shown in anticholinesterase-treated experimental animals.

A SFEMG investigation was made in 24 first-degree relatives of 12 patients with juvenile myasthenia gravis. Twenty-three of them had no history or clinical signs of myasthenia gravis or other neuromuscular disorder. One sister had experienced fatiguability during infections but the clinical investigation was inconclusive. SFEMG performed on EDC was abnormal in 8 of the relatives studied, one father, four mothers and three sisters, belonging to 7 of the 12 families. On average 5 out of 20 potential pairs showed increased jitter, 3 of these with intermittent blocking; about 25% of all recordings were abnormal, in contrast to about 75% in the clinically affected patients.[79,61]

Electrical Stimulation

In a number of patients the surface-recorded hypothenar muscle responses evoked by repetitive stimulation have been compared with the similarly evoked single fibre responses in abductor digiti minimi in an attempt to clarify the often encountered discrepancy between a normal or nearly normal study of surface responses and concurrently abnormal jitter recordings on voluntary activity.[39] The stimulus strength was submaximal for the nerve but maximal for the axons under study. Precautions were taken to make sure that the results of the study were not due to recruitment of new motor axons on repetitive stimulation.

In the SFEMG recording the number of action potentials from different muscle fibres has been compared in the first and fourth responses. In all cases the total number of responses decreased in proportion to the amplitude decrement in the simultaneous surface recording. However, this was often the net result of the disappearance of a number of responses and recruitment of action potentials from other muscle fibres from the second to the fourth stimulus (Fig. 79). Thus, lack of

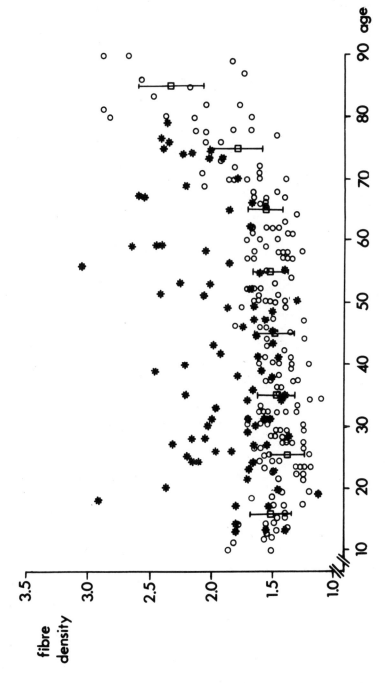

Fig. 78 Fibre density of motor units in the EDC muscle in treated and untreated patients with myasthenia gravis (asterisks). Each open circle is the fibre density for one healthy subject from our normal material (mean and SD for each decade is indicated). Note the increased fibre density in many myasthenic patients.

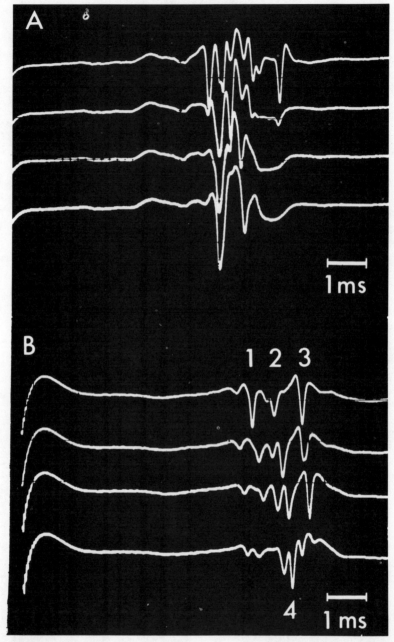

Fig. 79   Repetitive stimulation in myasthenia gravis. In A there is blocking of several
components with 2 Hz stimulation. In B there is blocking of fibre 1 after the
first stimulus, fibre 2 does not block, fibre 3 blocks only with the fourth
response, and fibre 4 is recruited with the second stimulus.
(From Schwartz and Stålberg, 1975)

surface decrement could be due to cancelling the effect of the disappearance of some fibres from the response by the new appearance of other fibres.

In many recordings the latency variability between stimulus and response was significantly increased although electrical stimulation tended to show more fibres with normal jitter than did voluntary activation; the difference was greater than could be explained by the fact that with electrical stimulation only one motor end-plate is involved at each jitter measurement compared with two on voluntary activation. Submaximal electrical stimulation introduces a bias towards large motor neurones, which is precisely opposite to voluntary activation. It appears that motor end-plates formed by large motor neurones tend to have a higher safety factor.

MYASTHENIC SYNDROME (EATON-LAMBERT SYNDROME)

In the myasthenic syndrome the jitter is considerably increased.[38,37,26] The maximal jitter values (MCD) can reach 500 μs and the interpotential interval range of 50 discharges can be up to 2000 μs. An impression is gained that the first impulse blocking occurs at generally higher jitter values than in myasthenia gravis. In the myasthenic syndrome the degree of blocking and jitter abnormality decreases with increasing innervation rate, the reverse of the finding in myasthenia gravis. The likelihood of blocking is also dependent on the preceding interval, so that with intervals in the physiological range (50–200 ms) a long interval is more likely to be followed by block than a shorter one. Tensilon sometimes has a long-lasting effect on the jitter and blocking, also seen in surface recordings[26]. The fibre density has been slightly increased in the cases of which we have had experience. This is in accordance with the finding of type II fibre grouping in the patients with type II fibre atrophy,[26] and may possibly reflect functional denervation similar to that seen after experimental botulinum intoxication (Duchen and Strich, 1968).

BOTULINUM INTOXICATION

In the patients with botulinum intoxication investigated with single fibre electromyography, increased jitter and blocking have been observed.[34] In cases in which fibre density has been measured the value has been lower than normal (J.R. Daube, personal communication). This is probably due to drop-out of fibres from the motor unit in a muscle in which no reinnervation has taken place.

It should be noted that the measured fibre density value also tends to be underestimated whenever there is impulse blocking (for example in untreated myasthenia gravis with many motor end-plates completely blocked).

TETANY

The distinguishing feature of tetany is spontaneous activity of muscle fibres potentiated during ischaemia or hyperventilation. It is believed to be generated presynaptically. As is known from CNEMG studies, spontaneous activity consists mostly of biphasic and some polyphasic motor unit-like potentials, often firing repetitively as so-called doublets, triplets and multiplets.

In SFEMG recordings[76] most of the spontar.cous activity recorded during tetanic cramps was found to appear in the form of single muscle fibre action potentials, with a few pairs and occasional triple potentials. The primary discharge was often followed by one, two or several extra-discharges. The intervals to the extra-discharges ranged considerably, from 4 to more than 10 ms. When the interval was below 10 ms, the action potential amplitude was decreased and the rise-time increased. There was considerable variation of consecutive intervals to the extra-discharge (an order of several hundred μs, MCD), and the firing rate of the primary discharge was slightly or moderately irregular. Due to the changed action potential amplitude and shape in the extra-discharge, the doublet may be mistaken for discharges of a pair of muscle fibres with large jitter. Closer inspection will then reveal interval-dependent changes in amplitude and steepness of the rising slope (Fig. 80) as in other extra-discharges (pages 61 and 80). At very short intervals, 4 to 5 ms, the action potential may become triphasic or even "disintegrated". Similar repetitive extra-discharges were also seen to follow voluntary discharges; they closely resembled the extra-discharges occurring in muscular dystrophies and polymyositis. Spontaneously firing potentials could also be recruited voluntarily.

Some action potentials, both voluntary and spontaneous, showed slight inflection of the fast rising slope, but otherwise corresponded to the criteria for single fibre action potentials. The significance of this deformation is not known; it may reflect an abnormality in membrane depolarization.

Other SFEMG parameters tended to be normal in patients with tetany, except for an occasional finding of slightly increased jitter in a small percentage of muscle fibre pairs.

MYOTONIA

The typical finding of high frequency discharges on concentric needle EMG makes the diagnosis of this group of disorders relatively simple. The effects of muscle percussion, of electrical stimulation, of cooling and of voluntary contraction help in the further differentiation of individual types of myotonia. The SFEMG gives additional information as to the microphysiology of the motor unit in these disorders and the findings are here briefly summarized.

Dystrophia Myotonica

This is the most common of the myotonic disorders. Spontaneous activity is less pronounced in SFEMG recording than in concentric needle EMG, probably because of the construction of the electrode. When recording with a concentric needle electrode mechanical activation of the muscle fibres is produced with the recording surface itself, which is at the tip, whereas in the SFEMG needle the tip is several millimetres away from the recording surface(s). The fibrillation potentials are single fibre action potentials and the high frequency discharges also consist of single fibre action potentials. The shape of the action potentials at high frequency discharges changes continuously, with an initial shortening followed by a prolongation of the rise time and sometimes the appearance of an extra notch. There is a parallel change of the amplitude of the action potential, initially an increase and then a decrease, sometimes to less than one half of the original amplitude.

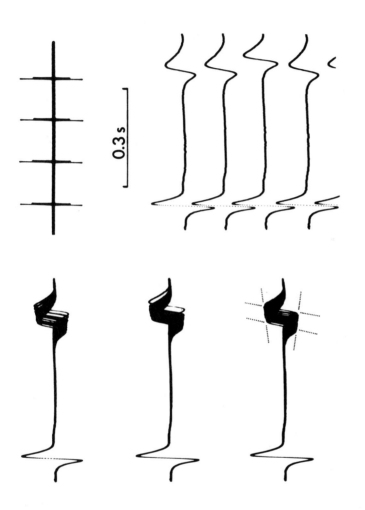

Fig. 80 A recording of spontaneous activity in a patient with tetany during hyperventilation. The second potential is an extradischarge with interval-dependent changes in amplitude and steepness of the rising slope (a "doublet").

Extra-discharges appearing 4–15 ms after the original discharge are frequently seen. If, in a multispike recording, the time interval to the extra-discharge is rather short, about 4 ms, it sometimes happens that not all of the components are seen in the extra-discharge. This is due to refractoriness in some of the muscle fibres giving rise to the original multispike action potential. As in all extra-discharges, the amplitude is systematically lower for short intervals, about 75% of the original or even less at 4 ms. The order of appearance of the individual components is usually the same in the extra-discharge as in the original discharge, indicating that the site of initiation is proximal to the terminal arborisation of the motor axon.

The fibre density is usually abnormal and can be considerably increased, particularly in clinically involved and atrophic muscles (Fig. 82). In general the fibre density increase is more pronounced in the EDC muscle than in the biceps brachii. The jitter is increased in dystrophia myotonica in about 25% of the recordings (Fig. 82). In a few recordings the jitter is less than normal, which is taken as an indication of fibre splitting.

Myotonia Congenita

Except for the myotonic activity concentric needle EMG is usually normal. In SFEMG recordings the myotonic discharges consist of single fibre action potentials which can be very similar to those described for myotonic dystrophy (page 132). At the highest discharge rates the shape may change, with a prolongation of the rise time and reduction of the amplitude. The fibre density is usually normal. The jitter is slightly increased in about 10% of the recordings and some blockings may appear. In one patient with very pronounced clinical myotonia the jitter was increased in 50% of the potential pairs studied. These relatively normal findings are in accordance with the usually normal histological findings in this disorder (Coërs and Woolf, 1959).

Paramyotonia Congenita

In this disorder the spontaneous activity may be initiated presynaptically, as two or three muscle fibres probably belonging to the same motor unit are activated simultaneously.[30] Another possibility is ephaptic activation of one muscle fibre by another. This is seen in cases of denervation (page 99) and might also be possible in myotonia, with its increased excitability. The myotonic activity starts during voluntary activation and can then continue for a long time. Sometimes one of the muscle fibres belonging to a group of muscle fibres with spontaneous activity suddenly gives a short high frequency burst and then becomes silent. This is also seen after the injection of Tensilon, to which voluntarily activated motor end-plates in this disorder seem to be sensitive. Different types of regular single discharges or grouped trains of discharges are seen in the spontaneous activity. On voluntary activation the muscle fibre density is normal. The jitter is increased in 70% of the recordings, probably indicating a disturbed membrane function at the motor end-plate.

Neuromyotonia

Three cases of neuromyotonia, or Isaacs' syndrome, have been studied[76]. All showed muscle stiffness interfering with voluntary movement and abundant visible twitches of limb and other muscles resembling myokymia. On SFEMG there was an

A   B

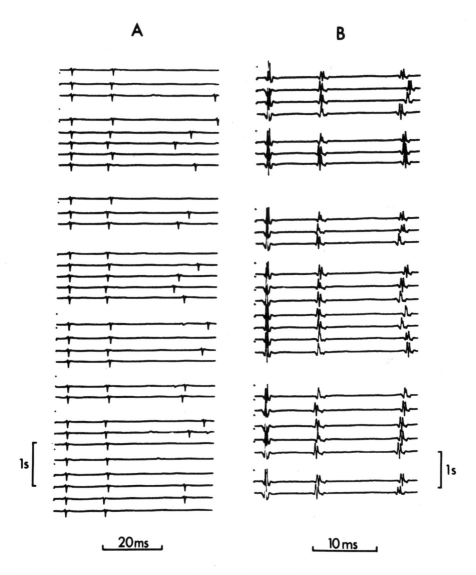

1s   1s

⌊__20ms__⌋   ⌊__10ms__⌋

Fig. 81 Recordings from two patients (A and B) with neuromyotonia. Triple
          discharges of a complex of muscle fibres are repeated at relatively low and
          moderately variable rate. The activity appears in clusters of variable
          lengths separated by resting periods of 0.5–1.5 seconds.

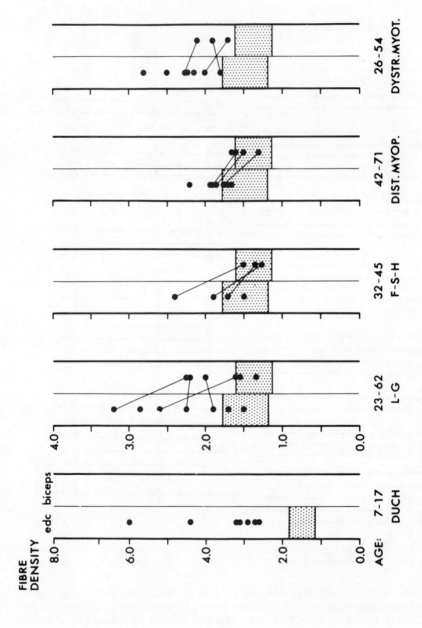

Fig. 82   Fibre density in EDC and brachial biceps muscles in different muscular dystrophies. Range of normal values (mean ± 2SD) is indicated as shaded areas. (From Stålberg, 1977)

abundance of spontaneous activity, sometimes appearing in complex patterns. The basic discharge consisted of one or several muscle fibre action potentials with jitter more than 5 μs. Typically, the basic discharge was repeated two or three times at moderately irregular intervals of about 4 to 10 ms (Fig. 81). Some spike components were often missing in the secondary discharges but sometimes new ones were recruited. The whole cycle recurred at irregular intervals (e.g. 2–10 per second), making up clusters of variable length separated by periods of 0.5 to a few seconds, which might be repeated indefinitely. Simpler patterns were also seen. Sometimes the basic discharge rate gradually increased to a point at which it stopped abruptly. After a few seconds the discharges were resumed at initially low but increasing rates and the whole cycle was repeated. The muscle fibres participating in spontaneous activity could also be recruited voluntarily. The spontaneous firing was enhanced during ischaemia, but stopped temporarily immediately after release of the tourniquet and after strong voluntary effort. In one patient blocking the ulnar nerve at elbow did not affect spontaneous activity in the hypothenar muscles, while blocking of the tibial nerve low in the popliteal fossa of another patient abolished almost all activity in the gastrocnemius muscle. Curarisation abolished all activity in the former patient. Diphenylhydantoin considerably reduced muscle stiffness and the recorded spontaneous activity.

Fibre density in voluntarily activated motor units was moderately increased in two of the three patients, and a proportion of muscle fibre pairs showed increased jitter and blocking.

Complexly patterned spontaneous activity closely resembling that described above was found in the thenar muscles in two cases of the carpal tunnel syndrome.

Pathological depolarisation in neuromyotonia thus originates in the nerve fibres, probably rather peripherally. In the cases of complicated discharge patterns there may exist more than one trigger point along an individual nerve fibre. The patterning depends on the recovery cycles of the individual trigger points.

MUSCULAR DYSTROPHIES

The first part of this section presents our findings in the commoner forms of dystrophies. This is followed by a discussion of ways in which SFEMG may contribute to further understanding of their pathophysiology.

DUCHENNE DYSTROPHY

A consistent finding in Duchenne dystrophy is an increase in fibre density, which in our series of patients was 3.5(2.6–6.0) in contrast with 1.45 in the normal muscle[60,44] (Fig. 82). Typical recordings with many muscle fibres within the uptake area of the electrode are shown in figure 83A. There are recordings with up to 14 spike components. The mean duration between the first and the last spike component in an action potential complex was 9 ms. The extreme value was 60 ms. Such a motor unit potential will alone give an interference pattern, as the first part of each discharge will appear before the last part of the preceding discharge at innervation rates higher than 15 per second (Fig. 84). In this situation it is impossible

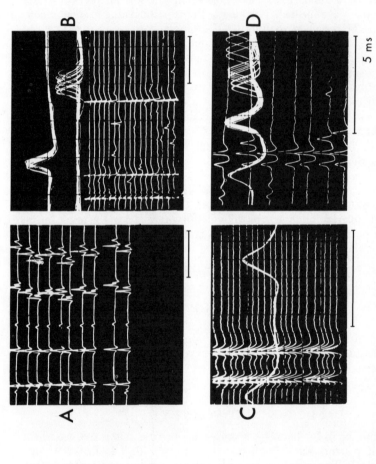

Fig. 83   Examples of SFEMG recordings from Duchenne dystrophy (A), limb-girdle dystrophy (B), facioscapulohumeral dystrophy (C), and distal hereditary myopathy (D). Note the large number of spike components in Duchenne (A). In A the late components show a common jitter, probably neurogenic. In B the jitter is within normal limits, for the second component 21 μs and for the third 43 μs. In C the jitter is small, 5 μs, indicating a split fibre recording. In D the first component has a normal jitter, 27 μs. The last component is blocking with a jitter of 131 μs. Time cal: 5 ms for "raster mode" display and 0.5 ms for the superimposed recordings. (From Stålberg, 1977)

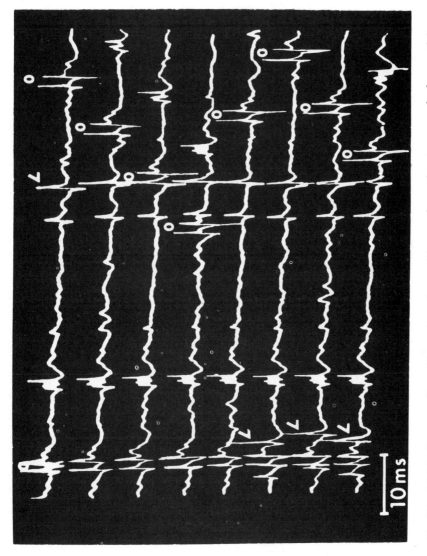

Fig. 84   Multispike recording, 50 ms, in a dystrophic muscle. o = start, ∠ = end of potential.

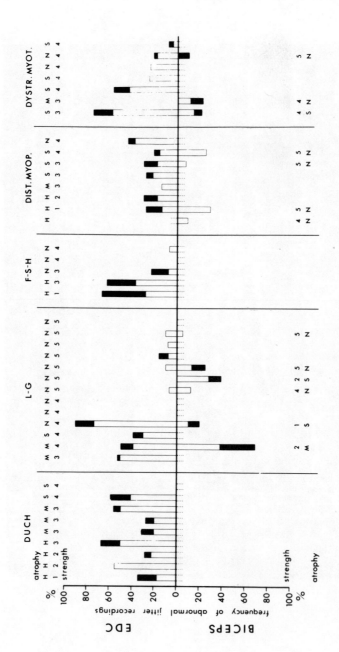

Fig. 85   Frequency of recordings with impulse transmission impairment in different muscular dystrophies. Increased jitter (normal value less than 0.3%) open area, impulse blocking black. Muscle not investigated is indicated with vertical dotted lines. Patients ranked according to decreasing muscular weakness and atrophy in each group. Degree of atrophy: N = no, S = slight, M = moderate, H = high. Strength classified according to the British Medical Research Council scale from normal (5) to no movements against gravity (1). (From Stålberg, 1977)

to determine the duration of the motor unit potential without triggering the sweep and using very low innervation frequencies; this applies even more to CNEMG, in which activity from many motor units is picked up at the same time. Even when recording a group of as many as 10 muscle fibres belonging to one motor unit of a weak muscle, 1–3 other motor units could commonly be recorded at the same time from the same site and with the same electrode surface at increasing strengths of contraction. This was not seen in the most severely affected muscles. In the late stages the fibre density may fall, but still be above normal. Moderately increased jitter was seen in about 30% of recordings in each muscle (Fig. 85). The later parts of the action potential complex in particular had a large jitter. Occasional blockings of single spike components were seen in about 10% of recordings with the largest jitter. In many of the patients studied there was concomitant blocking, i.e. two or more action potentials showing occasional synchronous blockings and a common increased jitter in relation to the rest of the complex. This transmission failure is most likely to be situated in the nerve twig[55] according to the explanation given in figure 30. In many recordings there is interdischarge interval-dependent jitter, especially for the later components, giving rise to pronounced simultaneous trends shown by components in the multispike potential ("the accordeon phenomenon"). This is an expression of strong velocity recovery function of the individual muscle fibres (page 74). Both slow trends and the short-term variability due to VRF should be taken into consideration when evaluating the jitter (page 41).

Propagation velocity was measured in a limited number of muscle fibres. The mean velocity in these recordings was slightly lower than in the normal material (Fig. 86). Propagation velocity was generally lower for the later spike components than for earlier ones in compound action potentials (Fig. 87).

Some insertions were followed by spontaneous rhythmic activity, usually appearing as complexes of action potentials with low MCD values between the individual spikes. The frequency could initially be as high as fifty discharges per second, but gradually declined to zero after some tens of seconds or stopped abruptly (c.f. "pseudomyotonia" or "bizarre high frequency discharges" in concentric needle EMG). Sometimes voluntarily discharging muscle fibres, on exceeding a certain discharge rate, suddenly started a pseudomyotonic discharge. Double discharges were sometimes recorded. Exceptionally, the single fibre action potentials in a multispike recording appeared in a different and changing order as compared to that in the original discharge (Fig. 49). This is interpreted as a sign of a very peripheral initiation of the extra-discharge in two or more terminal branches. The motor unit is then activated by axon reflexes starting antidromically from the point of initiation (see page 151).

The findings described above have also been obtained in muscles with very slight clinical involvement and a muscular strength rated normal on clinical testing. Two boys who later developed the disease were investigated at a preclinical stage below the age of 5 years. Both showed increased fibre density and many abnormal potential pairs with blocking.

Some carriers have shown abnormalities on SFEMG examination, particularly an increased MISI, but the changes have been of moderate degree.

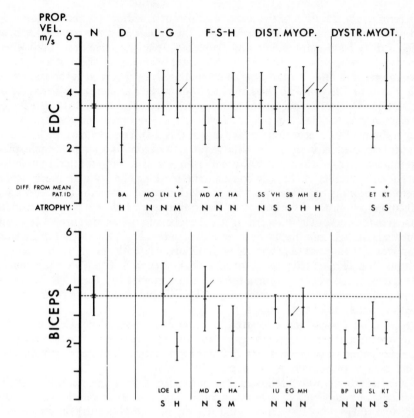

Fig. 86   Propagation velocity (mean, SD) in muscle fibres (N = 10–20) in EDC and
brachial biceps muscles as compared to normal values (mean, SD and SE
indicated, n = 200 for EDC and n = 443 for biceps). Significant (p < 0.01)
difference from mean indicated with + or −. Degree of clinical atrophy
indicated as N = no, S = slight, M = moderate, H = high. In some patients
(arrows) the range of velocity values exceeds that in normal muscles.
(From Stålberg 1977).

LIMB-GIRDLE DYSTROPHY

The fibre density is increased in this condition also, though usually not as much as
in Duchenne dystrophy. The mean number of the recorded fibres per electrode in a
series of 16 patients was 2.1 (range 1.5–3.2) in EDC[60] and 1.9 (range 1.4–2.3) in
biceps brachii[44] (see Figs 82, 83). The mean duration of the multiple spike potentials
was also increased (4 ms), but again less than in the Duchenne cases.

The jitter was increased in an average of 54% of the recordings in clinically weak
muscles (Fig. 85). Blockings occurred in less than 10% of the recordings, on average
in 4%. In one case with pronounced symptoms, 20% of the recordings showed
abnormal jitter, and 10% partial impulse blocking. In addition, concomitant blocking

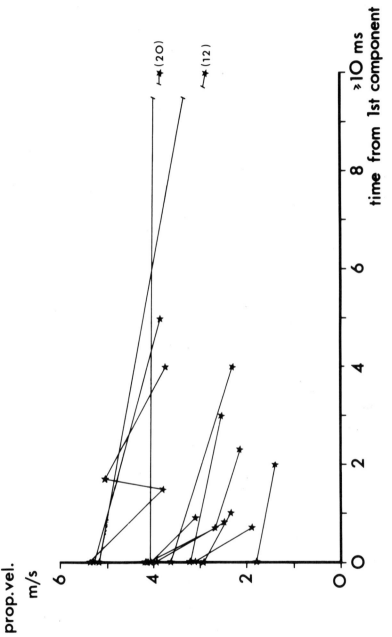

Fig. 87 Propagation velocity for the single muscle fibre components in double or multispike recordings. The late components have generally lower velocity than the early. Recordings from EDC in Duchenne dystrophy (From Stålberg, 1977)

was observed in some recordings. Seldom, but more frequently than in the normal muscle, were jitter values of less than 5 μs obtained. Spontaneous activity of the type found in the Duchenne cases was not observed in these patients. The abnormal findings were present in most muscles, including those with excellent strength.

FACIOSCAPULOHUMERAL DYSTROPHY

The findings in this disorder were similar to those in patients with limb-girdle dystrophy[44] (Figs. 82, 85 and 86).

GENERAL COMMENTS ON SFEMG FINDINGS IN MUSCULAR DYSTROPHIES

The findings obtained with the single fibre needle in the muscular dystrophies do not form patterns pointing to specific diagnoses. They provide information concerning transmission in different parts of the motor unit and the rearrangement of muscle fibres within the motor unit. The motor unit has a restricted repertoire of response to disease, and it is likely that most of the CNEMG and SFEMG parameters reflect relatively late dystrophic changes, either the drop-out of active fibres in the motor unit or compensatory changes, reinnervation and regeneration.[44]

The question raised in recent years — most pressingly by McComas (for a review see McComas, 1977) — as to whether the electrophysiological phenomena associated with certain myopathies are primary or are secondary to a neural disorder is still to some extent sub judice. This need not influence the interpretation of our SFEMG findings in the dystrophies, which is based on physiological principles worked out in normal subjects and, indeed, in known neurogenic disease. The SFEMG findings do not point to the site of the primary fault but illustrate functional disturbances and, to some extent, morphological changes in the periphery of the dystrophic motor unit.

Neuromuscular Transmission in Muscular Dystrophies

The *jitter* is often increased, slightly more in the group of Duchenne patients than in other muscular dystrophies. In the total material about 30% of the recordings in EDC and 20% in the biceps showed abnormal jitter, a third of which also showed intermittent impulse blocking. The jitter is usually more abnormal in the clinically more affected muscles and in patients reporting progression of symptoms during the past year. There tends to be a higher incidence of abnormal jitter in muscles with increased fibre density. In general the jitter is more pronounced in later components. Only exceptionally is paired blocking seen, interpreted as a sign of axonal impulse blocking. In a small proportion of action potential pairs the jitter is less than 5 μs, indicating a recording from a split muscle fibre. Usually the jitter does not change with changing mean discharge rate.

The site and nature of the observed impairment of impulse transmission is not yet established beyond doubt. At a certain stage of the disease process changes along the *degenerating muscle fibre* could lead to irregularities in impulse propagation before complete transmission failure takes place. Thus, in some recordings the degree of impulse blocking could be reduced by increasing the discharge rate, which might be explained by an increasing facilitation of impulse propagation (due to a supernormal phase of excitability during the recovery process) strong enough to overcome locally reduced excitability. Alternatively, the potentials recruited at higher innervation rates could be derived from ephaptically activated muscle fibres belonging to other motor units (pages 64, 101, 146). Not only focal lesions but general muscle fibre changes could cause impulse blocking. The cable parameters of the muscle fibre membrane are shown to be changed in some muscular disorders (Gruener, 1977) and could cause impaired impulse conduction. Another factor could be fibre atrophy leading to reduced propagation velocity in individual muscle fibres to a degree at which conduction failure occurs. The critical lower limit for propagation velocity value is not known. The muscle fibres showing intermittent impulse blocking did not in general show low propagation velocity values, but slowing of conduction at other sites cannot be excluded. The possibility of a myogenic jitter due to local or general factors needs to be further studied.

A second source of increased jitter and blocking could be disturbed *motor end-plate* function. Abnormalities of motor end-plate structure have been reported (Coërs and Woolf, 1959), with focal atrophy of the synaptic folds, but preserved acetylcholine receptors (Engel Mokri, Jerusalem, Sakakibara and Paulson, 1977). The jitter did not generally show any myasthenia-like changes with activity. Nevertheless in some of the cases in which Tensilon was tried transmission improved. This is not pathognomonic for motor end-plate failure, however, since the drug also has a positive effect on impaired impulse transmission along the terminal nerve twigs. The effect of Tensilon on muscle fibre impulse conduction is not known.

Thirdly, impulse transmission disturbances could be due to uncertain transmission in *regenerating* muscle fibres, which are formed from satellite cells.

Fourthly, impulse uncertainty is commonly seen in newly formed nerve sprouts and motor end-plates during *reinnervation*. In dystrophic muscle an innervation process is likely in connection with the maturation of satellite cells and the reinnervation of sections of muscle fibres separated by focal necrosis as well as with neurogenic denervation. Newly formed nerve sprouts and immature motor end-plates show transmission disturbances. In the normal muscle the jitter in the reinnervating motor units is normalised after 3–6 months. In dystrophic patients the increased jitter could indicate either continuous progression of the disease (the jitter was most abnormal in cases with clinical progression) or a slower functional maturation than in normal muscle of transmission in structures undergoing reinnervation or regeneration.

In some recordings an axonal block was strongly suspected because of concomitant blocking, but more often individual components showed blocking. This does not exclude the most peripheral parts of the nerve twigs, distal to the last branching point, as the site of impairment. Another finding indicating disturbed axonal impulse transmission was that the double discharges especially common in myotonic dystrophy were followed by a drop-out of the next normal discharge. As these double discharges activated the same group of fibres as were voluntarily activated and in the same sequence, the extra-discharge must be a neurogenic phenomenon. The failure of the next normal impulse cannot be explained by refractoriness of the muscle fibres, subnormality in the motoneurone cell, or impulse collision in the axon, but is most likely due to prolonged refractoriness of a weak point in the motor axon following peripherally elicited antidromic discharges or following the extra-discharges originating in the spinal cord. In one case (Duchenne) the extra-discharge was proved to start peripherally because the order of its spike components was reversed (page 83, Fig. 49).

Fibre Density in Muscular Dystrophies

The average *fibre density* in EDC was increased in all patient groups. The increase was generally less marked in biceps, where it was within normal limits in facioscapulohumeral dystrophy and in distal myopathy. In nearly all cases increased values were found in at least one of the muscles studied. There was no correlation between the fibre density and degree of atrophy, muscle strength or duration of disease. The *total duration* of the action potential complex and the MISI were increased, especially in Duchenne dystrophy. The values of the MISI were typically above 1 ms as compared with 0.2–0.6 ms in the normal muscle. Usually the spike components were well separated from each other in contrast to recordings in, for example, amyotrophic lateral sclerosis where the components were much more superimposed and the total duration shorter. There was also a tendency for the later components to have lower amplitudes, but this aspect is less pronounced than in chronic neurogenic disorders.

In some recordings, one or several new components were recruited into the action potential complex under study when the discharge rate was increased. When the rate was reduced these components disappeared again (page 64). This may be due to direct activation of adjacent inactive fibres belonging to other motor units by the action potentials from voluntarily activated fibres. Another possibility which cannot be excluded is an axonal block overcome by increased excitation at higher innervation rates.

The general finding of increased fibre density could theoretically be due simply to a general reduction of muscle volume because of *fibre atrophy* with local packing of muscle fibres in the motor unit, perhaps surrounded by fibrotic tissue. This explanation is rather unlikely since the fibre density was also increased in muscles in which no clinical atrophy was present. Simultaneous biopsy data are however lacking. As the volume conduction of the extracellular action potential depends on fibre diameter, atrophic fibres will be recorded over a shorter distance than fibres of normal size and therefore the effective uptake radius of the electrode will be reduced. The packing effect of atrophic fibres and the reduced recording radius are counteracting factors. This might explain why the fibre density in normal children below the age of 10 usually was only slightly higher than in normal adults in spite of a definite difference in fibre diameter. The fibre density in normal children was clearly lower than usually seen in adult patients with muscular dystrophy, although a child's arm circumference can be less than that of a patient with atrophy. However, excessive muscle fibrosis could theoretically either increase or decrease the recorded fibre density.

The effect of packing needs to be further studied, with direct correlation to biopsy data.

In a study of polymyositis it was shown that the fibre density value was not correlated to fibre diameter but to histochemical *fibre type grouping*.[27] In the present study the most likely explanation for the increased fibre density seems to be grouping

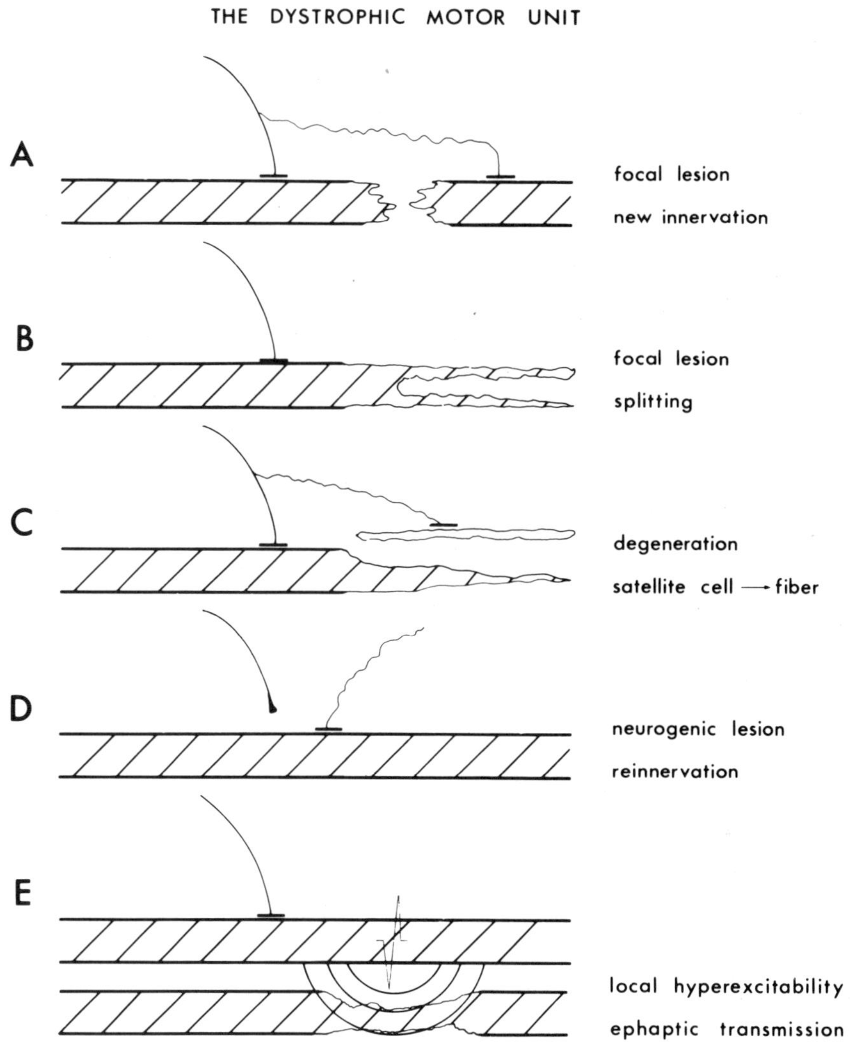

THE DYSTROPHIC MOTOR UNIT

Fig. 88 The possible explanations for the increased fibre density in muscular dystrophies. A: Focal lesion with segmental necrosis results in "myogenic denervation" of the distal part of the muscle fibre. This part may subsequently be reinnervated by a sprout from the same or another motor axon. B: following focal lesion, the remaining part of the muscle fibre may produce new buds, each giving rise to an action potential. C: Regeneration may take place by satellite cells producing new muscle fibres. The innervation is supplied from sprouts of existing axons. D: Partial loss of motor neurons, postulated by some authors, is followed by collateral sprouting to reinnervate the denervated muscle fibres. E: Muscle fibres of other motor units are, due to abnormal excitability, activated ephaptically by the action potentials of adjacent muscle fibres.

of muscle fibres belonging to the same motor unit (Fig. 88). However, this interpretation is not supported by the findings of Coërs. Telerman-Toppet and Gerard (1973) who reported mainly normal terminal innervation ratios (TIR) in facioscapulohumeral and limb-girdle dystrophies, with occasional increased values. Moreover, they found normal values in Duchenne dystrophy, in which condition our fibre density values were the highest. Moderate type grouping is however often seen in Duchenne (K. Engel, K.-G. Henriksson, personal communication).

The finding of increased fibre density in muscular dystrophies could be due to new innervation of parts of muscle fibres sequestered by focal transverse lesions as has also been suggested by Desmedt and Borenstein (1976). Furthermore, it could be due to new innervation of a regenerating muscle fibre developed from satellite cells. A third possibility is splitting of muscle fibres as a degenerative or regenerative phenomenon.

Fibre splitting is a common histological finding in muscular dystrophies, but is also seen exceptionally in normals. In this situation the jitter is below 5 μs, and a small proportion of the jitter in dystrophic muscle is in this range. The question arises as to whether a dystrophic split fibre always has a low jitter. If not, an excessive fibre splitting may contribute to the SFEMG finding of increased fibre density and to the signs of histochemical fibre type grouping.

A fourth explanation might be reinnervation of muscle fibres which had lost their functional innervation due to pre- or postsynaptic abnormalities.

Finally, a theoretical reason for increased fibre density value might be recruitment of adjacent fibres from other motor units by the mechanism of ephaptic transmission. This should give no correlation to type grouping or TIR.

The increased fibre density could thus indicate rearrangements of the motor unit due to abnormal innervation, preceded by myogenic or neurogenic lesions (Fig. 89). The total number of muscle fibres in the motor units is not generally increased as in classical neurogenic lesions, and this is indicated by the finding of normal or small surface-recorded motor unit potentials (for technique see page 31). This is in accordance with reports on motor unit size by McComas, Sica and Campbell (1973). It must be borne in mind however, that the amplitude of the motor unit potential is influenced not only by the number of muscle fibres but also by their diameters and probably also by the amount of muscle fibrosis and fatty replacement.

The generally lower fibre density in biceps than in EDC remains to be explained, though in distal myopathy the reason is obvious. In proximal dystrophies, in which the biceps is usually among the more severely affected muscles, the comparatively low fibre density may indicate that it is less able to achieve regenerative compensation.

POLYMYOSITIS

The patients studied include children and adults with "pure" polymyositis, dermatomyositis and polymyositis associated with collagen or malignant disease. The SFEMG picture differed little among these categories, but differed considerably from one patient to another and even in the same patient from one investigation to the next, depending on the stage at which the investigation was made.[27]

In the earlier stage, the fibre density is usually only slightly or moderately increased. The jitter is increased in most components and blockings are frequently

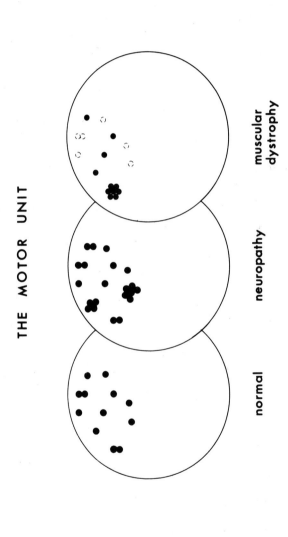

Fig. 89 Schematic explanation of arrangement of muscle fibres in the motor unit in different conditions.

seen. In some recordings there is concomitant blocking, probably a sign of impaired nerve conduction in newly formed sprouts. Some recordings show a larger jitter without blocking than is typical for ordinary neuromuscular block. This might be attributed to disturbed conduction either in the nerve twig or along the muscle fibre. In some recordings the jitter is smaller than normal, indicating a recording from a split muscle fibre.

Sometimes the degree of blocking increases during continuous activity, particularly in potentials with initially increased jitter and intermittent blocking. This is sometimes correlated to clinical fatiguability.

Later the fibre density is increased, and may be very high in nonprogressive phases of the disease. Here the jitter is less abnormal and blockings are only rarely encountered. There seems to be an inverse relationship between fibre density and atrophy. Patients with high fibre density tend to have less atrophy than patients with less increased fibre density, when atrophic changes may be pronounced. Atrophic muscle with lower fibre density may have a reduced capacity for effective regeneration and reinnervation. The increased fibre density might indicate reinnervation following an earlier denervation due to involvement of peripheral nerve twigs, or, more likely, following myogenic loss of innervation due to focal necroses along the muscle fibre. The part of a muscle fibre disconnected from its motor end-plate will behave initially as a denervated muscle fibre with fibrillation potentials (typical of active polymyositis) and will be reinnervated by its own motor unit or by a nerve twig from a neighbouring motor unit. The same holds true of newly formed muscle fibres.

Increased fibre density could also be caused by muscle fibre splitting, a phenomenon not uncommonly seen in polymyositis. However, in this case the jitter should be less than 5 μs (provided that conduction along muscle fibres is normal), which is true in only a small number of recordings. Increased fibre density is correlated to fibre type grouping in the histochemical investigation.

Double discharges of the whole action potential complex are frequently seen in polymyositis and are another sign of neural involvement since they indicate abnormal impulse generation in the nerve tree, probably peripherally.

The mean total duration of multiple spike potentials increases as recovery proceeds, mainly due to the adoption of new components. In the intermediate stages of the disease the multiple potentials may resemble those obtained in cases of Duchenne dystrophy and the MISI value may be as much increased, although the initial part of a multiple potential always has shorter inter-spike intervals in polymyositis than in Duchenne dystrophy, the early spikes being partly superimposed on one another. As recovery continues, the total duration of multiple potentials is shortened and the MISI value decreases. SFEMG can be used to support the diagnosis of polymyositis, but one should be aware that the findings can overlap with those in other diseases, especially the muscular dystrophies. The proportion of recordings with abnormal jitter, especially the proportion and degree of blocking, and to a lesser extent the duration values (total duration of multiple potentials and MISI), reflect and may be used to monitor the activity of the disease process and the effectiveness and extent of reparation. In doing so they shed light on the dynamics of the disease.

REFLEX STUDIES

Responses of single motor units in a variety of reflexes can be readily recorded by means of SFEMG. Studies of latency and latency variation (the reflex jitter) can be made with the oscilloscope sweep triggered by the stimulus. The magnitude of the jitter depends on the type of reflex, the main part being generated in the central portion of the reflex arc at the synapse, but there may be a significant contribution from the periphery, i.e. from receptors or afferent nerve fibres when these are stimulated electrically, from motor end-plates and sometimes, especially at high and irregular activation rates, from the muscle fibre and motor axon.[71,77,81] Single motor units are easily recognised by their all-or-nothing behaviour at threshold stimulation. When the recording is made from more than one motor unit, recognition is easier when the electrode is positioned so that the motor unit studied appears with more than one muscle fibre action potential. In latency and jitter studies the stimulus strength (pages 27 and 33) and degree of temporal dispersion of the afferent volley must be taken into account. In addition, the afferent and descending activity from other sources (e.g. respiration), as well as mental factors such as anxiety and distraction, may significantly influence the results. For the sake of convenience, we include here the axon reflexes and recurrent responses, even though they do not fulfil the criteria of a true reflex.

AXON REFLEXES

When electrical stimulation is performed with an electrode inserted in the muscle it is often possible to record single muscle fibre responses which show dual latency distribution, depending on stimulus strength. With a weaker stimulus the latency is longer, and on raising the strength to a certain value the responses "jump over" to an earlier latency. If the stimulus strength is kept at this value there is random alternation between the short and the long latency, but when it is further increased only short latency responses are obtained (Fig. 90 A–C). The phenomenon is explained as an axon reflex (Fig. 90 D) in which the weak stimulus does not directly activate the axonal branch belonging to the muscle fibre from which the recording is being made, but instead depolarizes another branch which is nearer (or has a lower threshold). The antidromically propagated nerve impulse then invades other branches giving rise to axon reflex responses. When the stimulus is made stronger, it activates the axonal branch to the observed muscle fibre directly, which results in a stepwise shortening of the latency.[59,80]

Axon reflexes of the type described can be obtained by stimulating the nerve proximal to the point at which it enters the muscle. The closer to the muscle stimulation is made, the better is the chance of recording axon reflexes, since most of the branching of motor axons occurs immediately proximal to the point at which the nerve enters the muscle and particularly inside the muscle. Axon reflexes are most easily elicited by stimulating inside the muscle near the motor point. "Jumps" of the latency between the direct and axon reflex response can range in different cases from

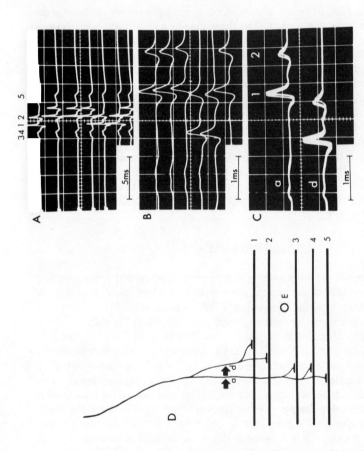

Fig. 90   Intramuscular electrical stimulation producing a complex response of action potentials from five muscle fibres, all of one motor unit, two of which (1 and 2) respond with two latencies, whereby they are always linked together. Note different time calibrations in A and B–C. In C, 7 discharges were superimposed with each of the two latencies, to show the relative constancy of both latencies. D, schematic explanation of this phenomenon based on an axon reflex. The two fibres with dual latency are activated either directly through their own axonal branch (d) or, when the stimulus is subthreshold, through the branch to the other three fibres in the recording via an axon reflex arc (a). In this case the antidromically propagated impulse invades the branch to fibres 1 and 2, and the response appears with a longer latency (From Stålberg and Trontelj, 1970).

a few hundred to a few thousand μs. Sometimes the same axon reflex can be activated by another stimulating electrode at a more proximal point. In this case conduction velocity can be calculated for both branches and, by extrapolation, the location of the branching point can be estimated. In some normal subjects such calculations suggested axonal branching considerably higher than one would expect from histological studies (Kashef, 1966; Wray, 1969). In one case branching was located in the tibial nerve as high as 10–15 cm above the gastrocnemius muscle,[59] and in another case of an axon reflex recorded in the orbicularis oculi the branching was estimated to occur in the intracranial portion of the facial nerve.[80]

In cases of reinnervation, axon reflexes can be recorded with longer latency changes and sometimes with more proximal branching points (Fullerton and Gilliatt 1965). In reinnervation of facial muscles a study of axon reflexes can demonstrate collateral branches of axons normally supplying another muscle. In such cases electrical stimulation over the supraorbital foramen may produce an axon reflex in the orbicularis oculi muscle from a frontalis motor neurone which may be indistinguishable from the first component of the blink reflex unless latency variation is studied[80] (see page 160).

Due to the mechanism of axon reflexes, abnormal impulses generated in the periphery of the axonal tree will activate the whole motor unit. For the same reason, it is also likely that the whole motor unit is activated even when one of the most peripheral axonal branches is stimulated with an intramuscular electrode. One type of fasciculation, extra-discharges, neuromyotonic activity, and also muscle cramps, may involve axon reflexes.

The jitter of the axon reflex responses is not greater than that of responses to stimulation of the direct axonal branch, provided that in both cases the stimulus is above threshold. Thus there is no latency variation added at the branching point. Care should be taken, however, in jitter studies made by intramuscular electrical stimulation, to recognize and exclude axon reflexes alternating with direct responses when the jumps are small.

F-RESPONSE

The F-wave, which is the late and variable response following the M-wave, especially in the distal limb muscles at supramaximal nerve stimulation, is now generally believed to be composed of recurrent discharges of antidromically activated motor neurones. With SFEMG it is possible to isolate muscle fibre action potentials with the same latency as the surface recorded F-wave. A single fibre F-response is always preceded by a short latency response from the same fibre (corresponding to the M-wave) so that when the M-response is missing on threshold stimulation, no F-response is present (Fig. 91 A). This indicates that responses of this type are indeed recurrent responses due to antidromic activation of the motor neurone.[72] At supramaximal stimulation, the F-responses of individual neurones appear randomly, following 0.1 to 20% of M-responses. From some motor neurones recurrent responses are not obtained. The frequency of appearance can be increased by a variety of manoeuvres (such as Jendrassik's) which presumably produce facilitation of the motor neurone pool. Conversely, it can be decreased by antagonistic muscle movement.[72] In some neurones with a high incidence of

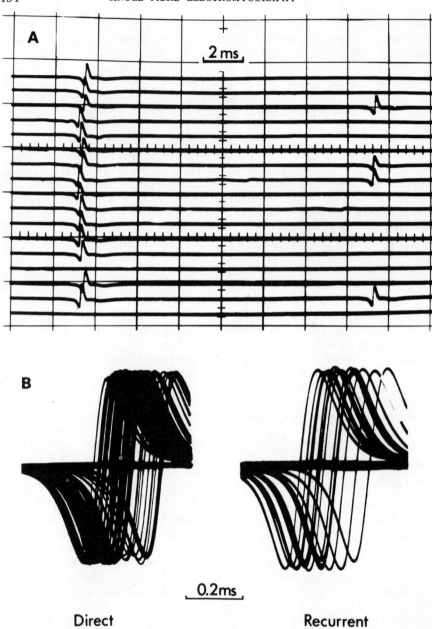

Fig. 91   Direct and recurrent responses of a muscle fibre in abductor pollicis brevis. A. If at threshold stimulus the direct response is missing, the recurrent response is also missing. B. The direct and recurrent responses of the same muscle fibre superimposed at higher sweep speed. The jitter is similar in both responses. (From Trontelj, 1973a)

F-responses at rest, voluntary activity in the recorded muscle may reduce the number of F-responses.

The latency variation of successive recurrent responses of individual muscle fibres is usually only slightly larger than that of the M-responses of the same fibres (1 : 1.3 in the average, Fig. 91 B).[71,72] The additional variation is due to the varying delay at the axon-soma junction. This is in sharp contrast to the markedly variable latency of the surface-recorded F-wave, which is due to activation of different populations of motor neurones by successive stimuli. F-responses are more abundant in spastic muscles, but have the same characteristics as described above.

H-REFLEX

The H-reflex appears in surface recordings as a late response on weak nerve stimulation when the M-response is small or absent. When the M-responses become larger with increasing stimulus strength, the H-responses are obliterated, which has been interpreted as being due to collision between antidromic and reflex impulse in the most proximal part of the motor axon (Diamantopoulos and Gassel, 1965). When recording is made from a single motor unit, the H-response is indeed seen to be obliterated when the stimulus is strong enough to depolarize the motor axon directly and give an M-response (Fig. 92 A).

However, in up to one third of the soleus motor neurones tested with series of 100 stimuli at 0.3 Hz, both an M and an H-response could occasionally be elicited by one and the same stimulus (Fig. 92 B), particularly if some method of facilitation was used[71] (In this case the late responses could be distinguished from recurrent responses by their larger latency variation). This suggests that here collision of the antidromic and reflex impulse in the motor axon cannot be the explanation for the obliteration of the H-reflex at higher stimulus strengths.

In SFEMG recordings the H-reflex, in contrast to the recurrent response, shows large latency variation.[67,69,71,73] The mean latency variation for 25 motor neurones was about 185 μs (SD) at threshold stimulus strength. When the stimulus strength was increased by half-way to the threshold for the M-response, the latency variation decreased to about 100 μs, while at threshold for the M-response it again increased to about 150 μs (Fig. 93 A and B). Mean latencies showed similar changes. At the threshold for the M-response, not only did the mean latency and latency variation increase, but some reflex responses failed to occur (Fig. 92 A). This may have been due to simultaneous stimulation of fast-conducting inhibitory fibres.

Manoeuvres facilitating the H-reflex will decrease the mean latency of the individual motor neurone responses by as much as 0.5 ms. Conversely, inhibitory manoeuvres can increase the mean latency.

The latency variation of the single fibre H-response includes the neuromuscular jitter and the variability in impulse initiation at the site of stimulation, as well as the variation in synaptic delay at the single ventral horn cell. The contribution of the first two factors can be estimated by measuring the M-response variation (usually less than 20 μs). This leaves between 80 and 150 μs to be attributed to the variation in the central synaptic delay when experimental conditions are kept as constant as possible.

With SFEMG recordings the surface recorded H-wave of the soleus has been shown to contain varying proportions of recurrent responses at stimulus strengths

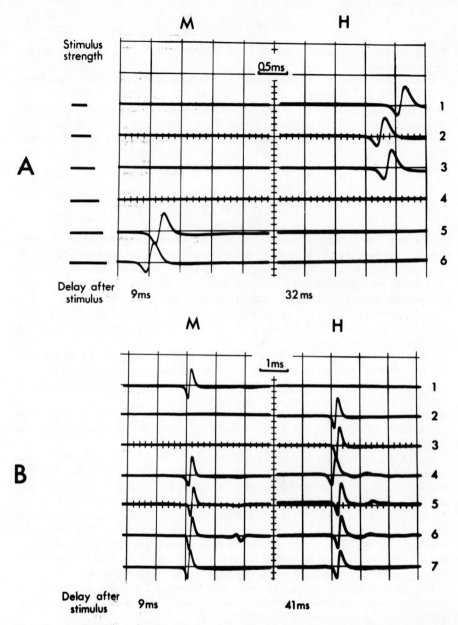

Fig. 92   A. Typical recording from a muscle fibre in the soleus activated by an increasingly strong stimulus to the tibial nerve. Each sweep is expanded twice, to show latency changes of both H and M-responses. The H-reflex responses are obliterated when the motor axon is depolarized directly giving a M-response. However, the H-reflex may be occasionally extinguished even before the appearance of an M-response in the same neurone (trace 4). B. Another soleus muscle fibre, activated by some of the stimuli (traces 4–7) both in the M and in the H-response (From Trontelj, 1971).

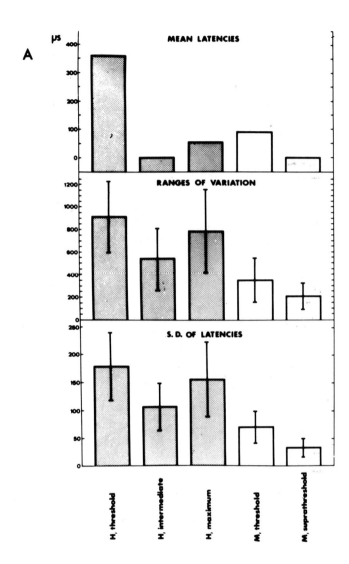

Fig. 93 A. Mean latency and latency variation of 25 soleus motor neurones in the
H-reflex at 3, and in the M-response, at 2 stimulus strengths. Maximum
strength is that at which about 50% of H-reflex responses are replaced by
direct responses and intermediate is mean of maximum and threshold
strengths. Mean latencies are expressed as increase in reference to the value
obtained at intermediate (H) and suprathreshold (M) stimulus strengths,
respectively (From Trontelj, 1973a).

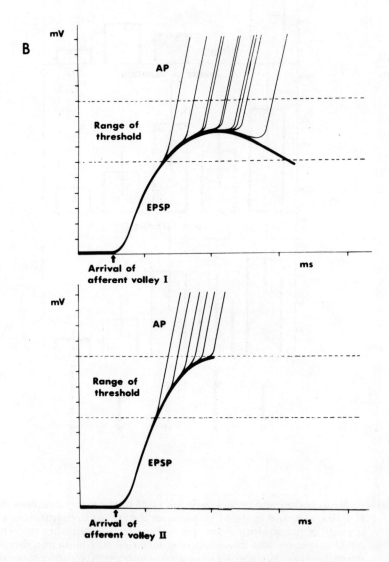

Fig. 93   B. Schematic explanation of latency variation in H-reflex at threshold and
         higher stimulus strength (From Trontelj, 1973b)

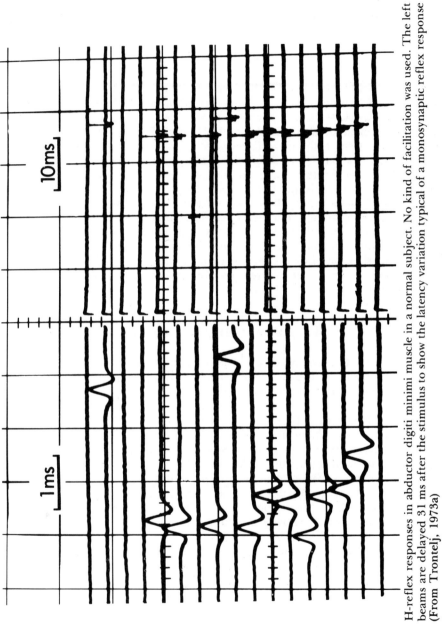

Fig. 94 H-reflex responses in abductor digiti minimi muscle in a normal subject. No kind of facilitation was used. The left beams are delayed 31 ms after the stimulus to show the latency variation typical of a monosynaptic reflex response (From Trontelj, 1973a)

above the threshold for M-response. Similarly, the surface-recorded F-wave of distal limb muscles contains a few H-reflex responses, (Fig. 94) particularly if some kind of facilitation be used[72] (cf. Hagbarth, 1962) or in spasticity.

BLINK REFLEX

The electrically evoked and surface-recorded blink reflex has two components. With SFEMG recording, successive responses of individual motor neurones in the first component show a latency variation which is about 2.5 times larger (about 400 μs at supra-threshold stimulus) than that of the H-reflex (Fig. 95).[82,83,84] On increasing the stimulus strength the mean latency decreases more than in the case of the H-reflex, but the latency variation shows little change. Occasionally a bimodal distribution is found with a separation of peaks of about 5 ms. This suggests that at least one interneurone is involved.

The second component of the surface-recorded blink reflex commonly contains repetitive discharges of the same motor neurone, most often two, and up to seven.[81] The latency variation of the earliest discharges is of the order of 3000 μs (three times that of the first component) and increases for later components. The different components show an obvious common random latency variation. This seems to indicate that a part of the polysynaptic pathway is common for the different components.

FLEXION WITHDRAWAL REFLEX

The flexion withdrawal reflex of the lower limbs shows an even more complex surface response than the blink reflex. When recorded from single muscle fibres of the tibialis anterior responses may be repetitive, from two to about ten discharges per stimulus. There is no distinct first component as in the case of the blink reflex. The latency variation increases for successively later components. Their ranges overlap, and the number of components varies with successive stimuli.[74,77] These two factors make measurements of latency variation difficult. For the early components the variation is estimated at more than 7000 μs (Fig. 96). Again there is the phenomenon of parallel latency variation of individual motor neurone responses in different components. The larger latency variation in the second component of the blink reflex and especially in the flexion withdrawal reflex suggests a larger number of synapses in the central pathway as compared with the H-reflex and the first component of the blink reflex. It is unlikely, however, that there is a linear relationship between degree of latency variation and number of synapses. Repetitive discharges of interneurones and alternating central pathways probably contribute significantly to the total latency variation.

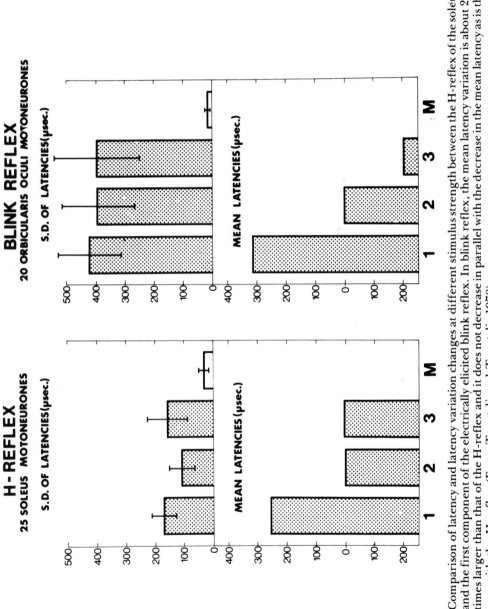

Fig. 95   Comparison of latency and latency variation changes at different stimulus strength between the H-reflex of the soleus and the first component of the electrically elicited blink reflex. In blink reflex, the mean latency variation is about 2.5 times larger than that of the H-reflex and it does not decrease in parallel with the decrease in the mean latency as is the case with the H-reflex (From Trontelj and Trontelj, 1978).

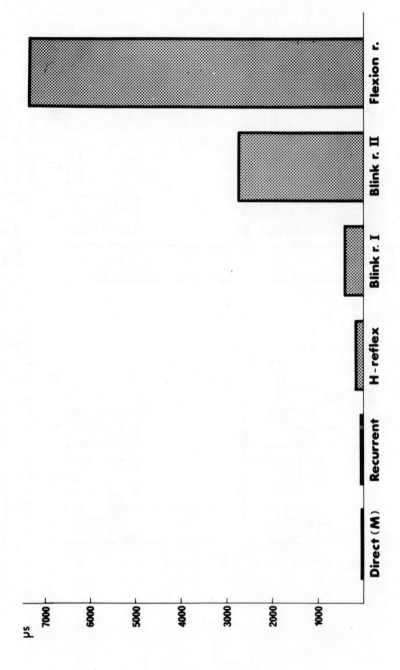

Fig. 96   Latency variation of some responses to electrical stimulation. M = direct responses, Blink r. I and II refer to the first and second component of the blink reflex. In the latter as well as in the flexion withdrawal reflex, the earliest responses were computed (From Trontelj, Trontelj and Stålberg, 1973).

PUDENDAL REFLEXES

Electrical stimulation of cutaneous and muscular afferents in the pudendal region gives rise to a variety of responses in the individual motor neurones.[75] Some have short latency and latency variation in the range of H-reflex values, while others have latency variations of various degrees, up to more than 5000 μs, and show repetitive discharges of individual neurones (Fig. 97). In contrast to the flexion withdrawal reflex, these responses frequently require higher stimulation rates (above 5 to 10 Hz) to be elicited, and are considerably more resistant to habituation.

TENDON JERK

The latency variation between the stimulus, the tendon tap, and the single fibre reflex response, corresponding to the surface-recorded T-wave, is usually larger than in the case of the H-reflex, even when the same motor neurones are compared.[77] Values as low as 200–300 μs are occasionally obtained, but the average is about 450 μs, with occasional values exceeding 1500–2000 μs. In these cases it is frequently possible to observe a bimodal distribution, with separation of the peaks by 2 to 4 ms and with parallel latency variation resulting in partial overlapping in nonsequential histograms (Fig. 98). By adding weak muscle vibration at 50–100 Hz the responses were seen more often in the later of the two ranges of values. During the postvibratory period, the shorter latency values were preferred (Fig. 99). This might indicate that a disynaptic pathway may sometimes be involved.

TONIC VIBRATION REFLEX (TVR)

A vibrator was designed which could make selected single pulses stronger than the background vibration. The vibratory pulses were rectangular in order better to define the mechanical stimulus. When the selected pulses (1 per 10–50 at 100 Hz) are made slightly stronger (by about 5%) than the background pulses, which are just subthreshold for the TVR, responses are obtained from single motor neurones to each stronger stimulus. Alternatively, the background pulses are dropped out, so that the vibrator acts as a tendon hammer. The latency variations are roughly similar in both situations (they tend to be somewhat larger during vibration), but the mean latency is usually 2–3 ms longer during vibration (Fig. 100). This seems to indicate that the TVR as elicited in this situation has a strong monosynaptic or at least oligosynaptic contribution.[74,77]

In addition to the responses described, the same motor neurones may discharge at intervals still time-locked to the stronger pulses, but with longer latency and much larger variation.

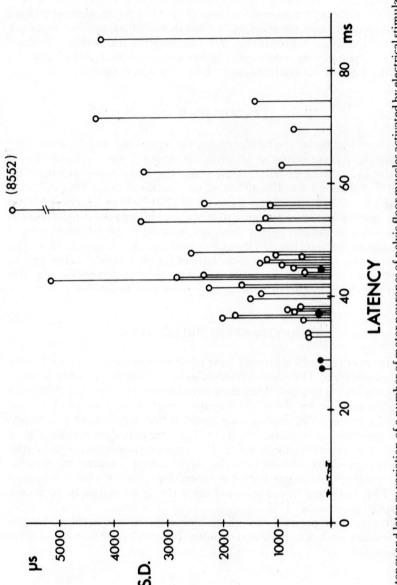

Fig. 97   Latency and latency variation of a number of motor neurones of pelvic floor muscles activated by electrical stimulation of the perineum. Dashes represent direct responses, full circles short-latency reflex responses with small variation (monosynaptic or oligosynaptic) and empty circles polysynaptic reflex responses with large latency variation (From Trontelj, Janko, Godec, Rakovec and Trontelj, 1974).

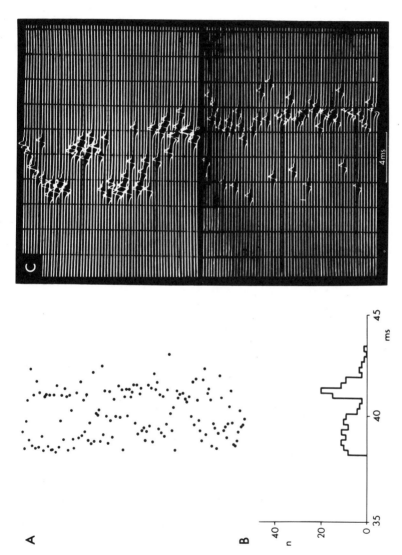

Fig. 98   Bimodal distribution of the latencies of a single muscle fibre in the tendon jerk. A sequential, B nonsequential histogram and C actual recording of another fibre. There is a parallel slow trend in both shorter and longer latencies resulting in partial overlapping in the nonsequential histogram (From Trontelj, Stålberg and Dimitrijević, 1978)

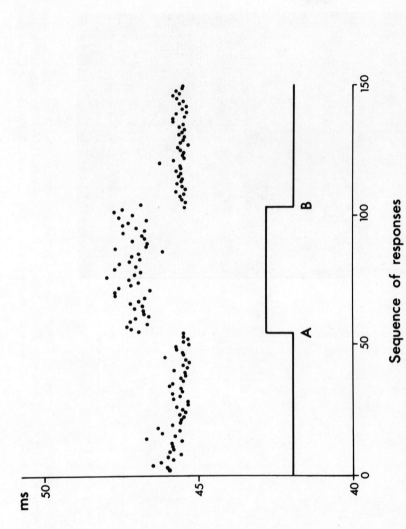

Fig. 99   Sequential histogram of the latencies of single muscle fibre responses in tendon jerk showing bimodal distribution. Weak vibration applied at A results in preference for the longer latencies. Withdrawal of vibration at B is followed by preference for the shorter latencies.

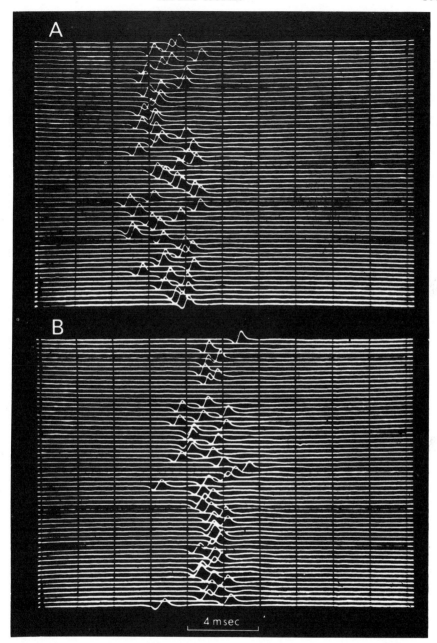

Fig. 100   A. Responses of a single quadriceps femoris muscle fibre to tendon taps at
2 Hz. B. The same muscle fibre driven by vibration at 100 Hz. The sweep is
now triggered by the 5% stronger vibration pulses occurring at a rate of 1
per 10 ordinary pulses (C see over). The responses in B have slightly
longer latency but comparable latency variation (From Trontelj, Stålberg
and Dimitrijevič, 1978)

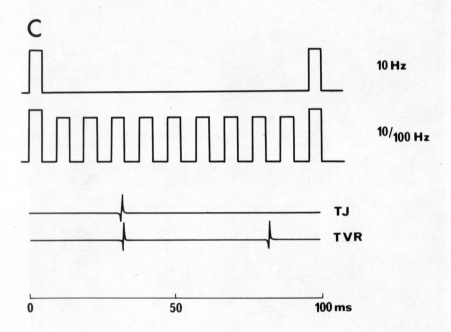

ATLAS

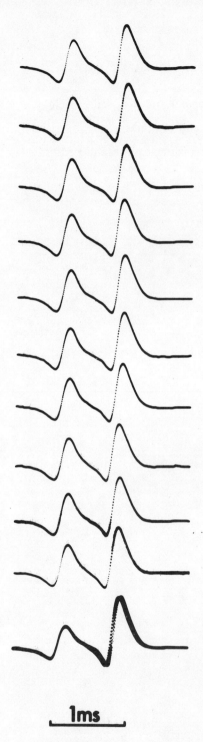

1ms

Fig. 1 a-b   Examples of normal action potential pairs.

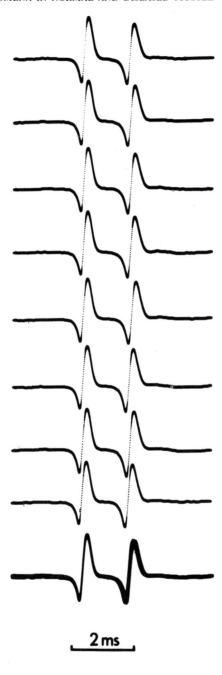

Fig. 1b

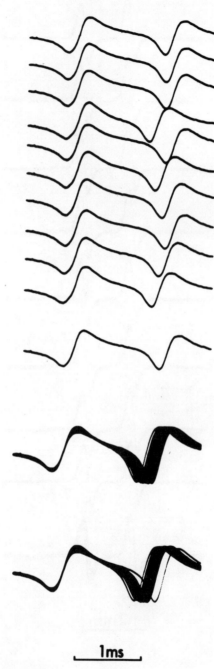

1ms

Fig. 2a-b Normal potential pairs
Fig. 2a potential pairs with jitter close to normal upper limit (MCD 46μs)

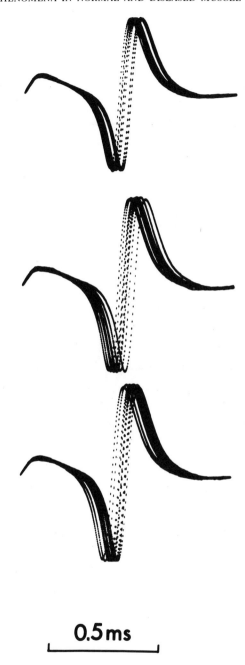

0.5 ms

Fig. 2b   Trigger on first action potential at beginning of sweep; delay has not been used.

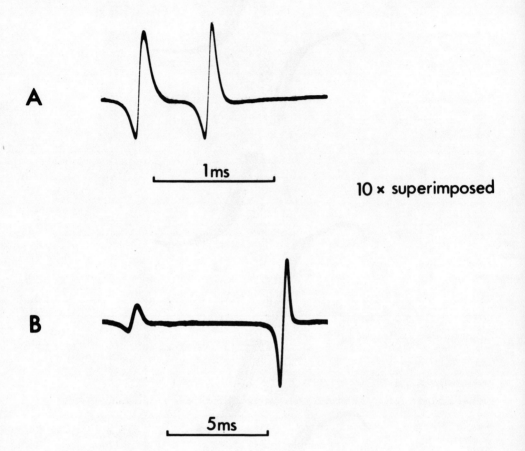

Fig. 3 Examples of action potential pairs with low jitter. A, in normal muscle; B, in a patient with muscular dystrophy.

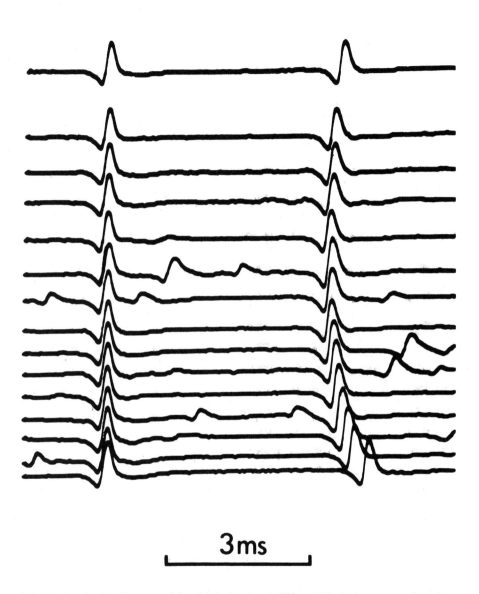

3ms

Fig. 4 A pair of action potentials with increasing MIPI at high discharge rate. A patient with limb-girdle muscular dystrophy.

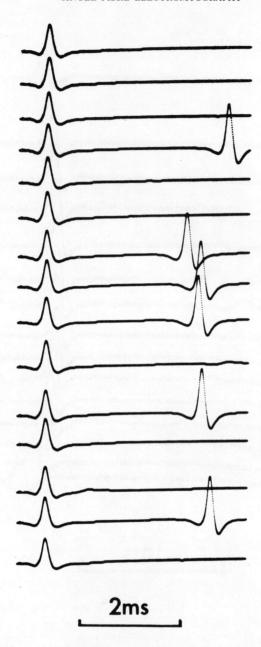

2ms

Fig. 5   A potential pair with increased jitter and blocking recorded from a quadriceps muscle of a healthy young adult. Out of 25 recordings in this subject only one showed this phenomenon.

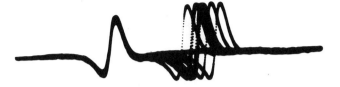

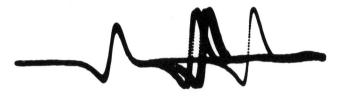

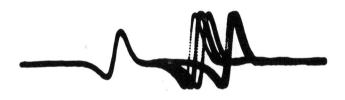

2ms

Fig. 6   A potential pair from extensor digitorum brevis muscle of a normal subject with increased jitter and partial blocking. Such findings are frequent in this muscle even in young normal subjects.

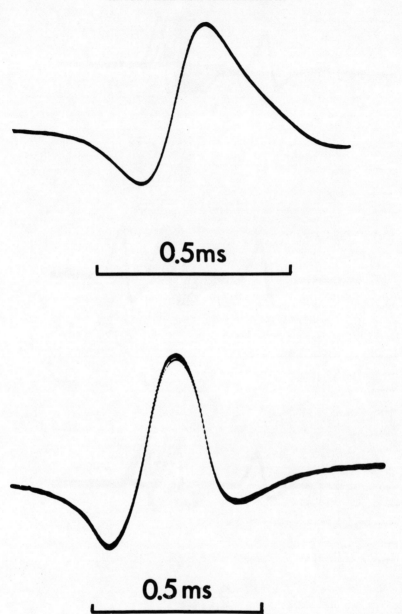

Fig. 7   Examples of action potential deformity (from a patient with tetany). There is no jitter between the different parts of the action potentials (15 discharges superimposed). Disturbed repolarization? Superimposition of another muscle fibre's action potential with low jitter?

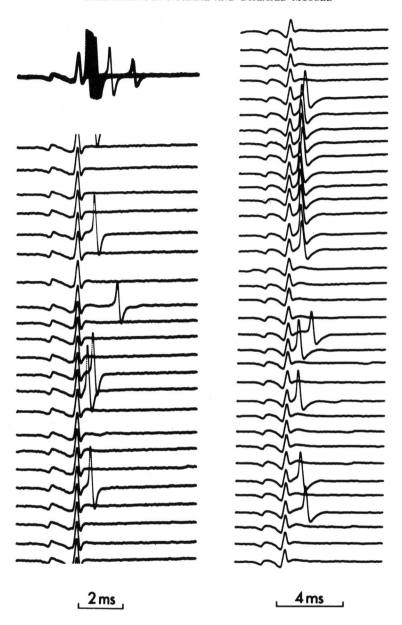

2 ms

4 ms

Fig. 8   False increased jitter and blocking due to recruitment phenomenon. The last action
potential shows large jitter and blocking, but also interpotential interval dependent
amplitude changes. At higher innervation frequencies the jitter and the delay of the
third potential become smaller.

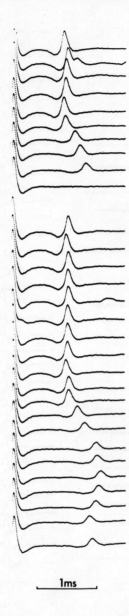

1ms

Fig. 9   Another example of the recruitment phenomenon in a normal subject. Such potentials
seem to be more frequent in the frontalis muscle. Notice gradual increase of the
amplitude and reduction of the jitter.
After a short pause in activity there is transient blocking, the amplitude decreases
again and the interval and jitter increase. After a long pause the second potential
is lost. In contrast to the previous example the polarity of the second potential is not
reversed.

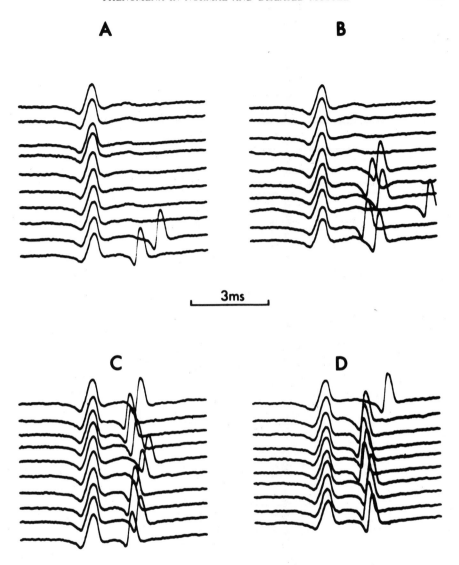

Fig. 10   Another type of the recruitment phenomenon. The recruited potential does not
show interpotential interval-dependent changes in the amplitude of the recruited
potential, but there is an inverse relationship between the degree of jitter and
frequency of blocking on the one hand and the discharge rate on the other hand
(compare A and D). At uniform discharge rate too the jitter shows a tendency to
decrease over a period of time.

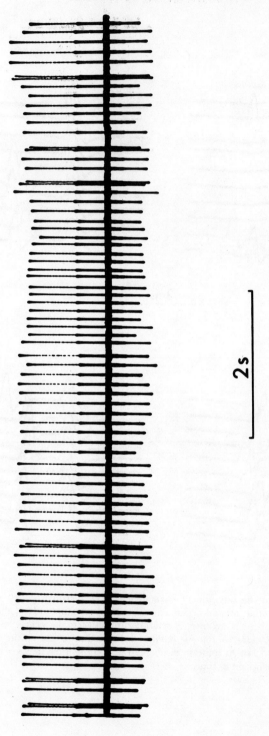

Fig. 11   A potential pair in voluntary activity with the phenomenon of double discharges. (Changes in amplitude are due to partial superimposition of spikes with jiter.) The extra-discharge prevents the occurrence of the next normal discharge. The site of generation must be distal to the motor neuron cell.

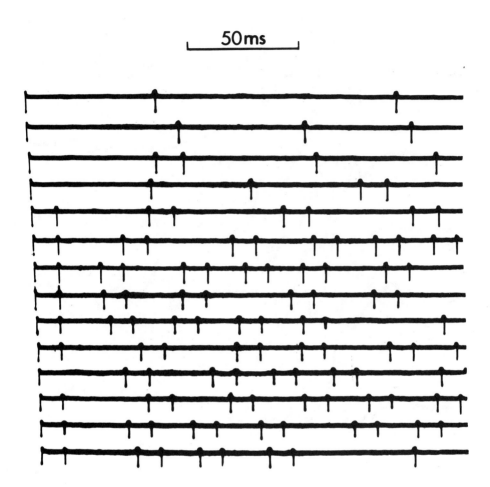

Fig. 12   Double discharges of a muscle fibre in a patient with Duchenne muscular dystrophy. The extra-discharges are quite regular above certain discharge rate (about 20 per second). The interval to the extra discharge varies between 10 and 12 ms.

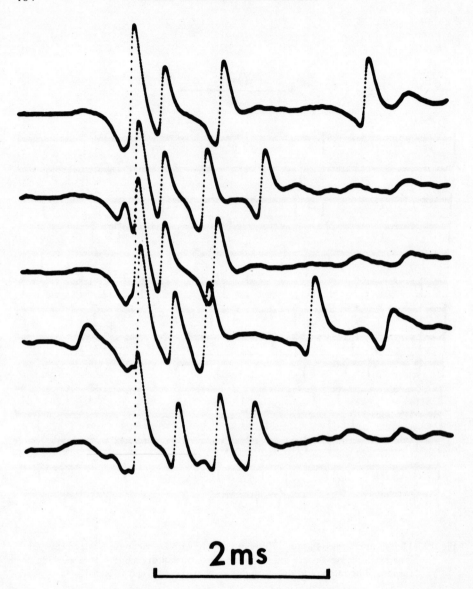

2ms

Fig. 13   A multispike potential with increased jitter and blocking obtained from extensor digitorum brevis muscle of a normal adult aged 20 years.

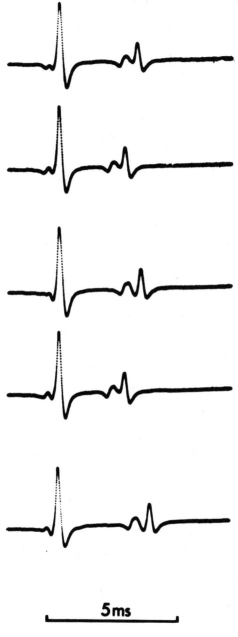

5ms

Fig. 14a

Fig. 14 A and B   Two examples of increased axonal jitter. This can only be identified when at least four muscle fibres are recorded.

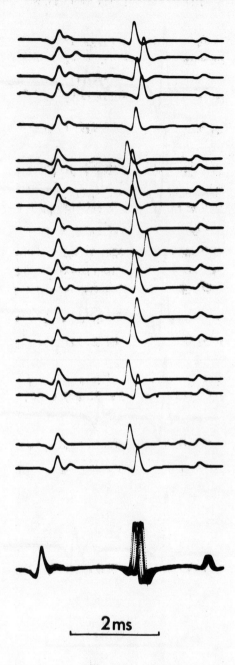

Fig 14b.

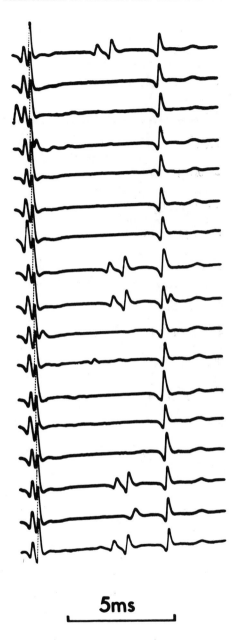

5ms

Fig. 15 Axonal blocking in a case of Duchenne muscular dystrophy. Potentials number 3 and 4 frequently block together and they also show increased jitter in relation to the rest of the complex.

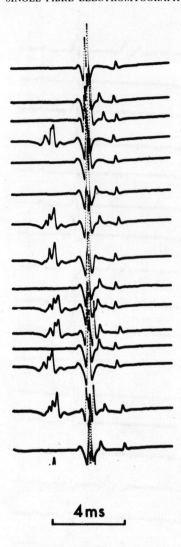

4 ms

Fig. 16   Another example of axonal blocking in a patient with syringomyelia. The unusual feature here is that the blocking part of the complex precedes the more stable part.

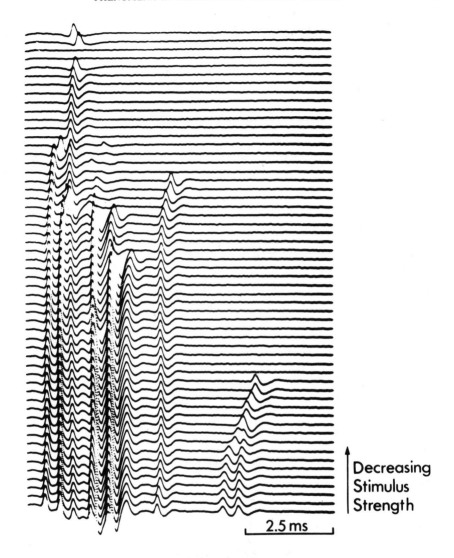

Fig. 17   Intramuscular stimulation in denervated muscle. Drop-out of individual spike components preceded by increase in latency.

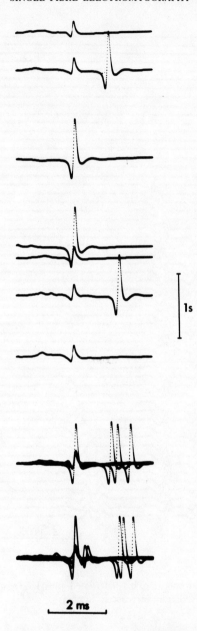

Fig. 18   Fasciculation potentials. Upper part with moving film to show the rather rapid
and irregular discharge rate. Below two groups of 10 superimpositions. The two
fibres appear independently or jointly, with variable interpotential intervals and
in changing order. A case of amyotrophic lateral sclerosis.

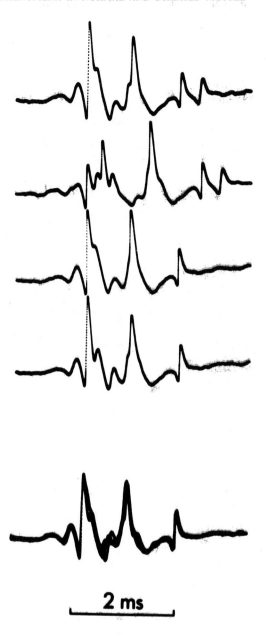

2 ms

Fig. 19   Another, more complex fasciculation potential of rather stable shape, with only moderate jitter and little variation in number of spikes. (The vertical spacing between the single traces does not represent interdischarge intervals.) Another patient with amyotrophic lateral sclerosis.

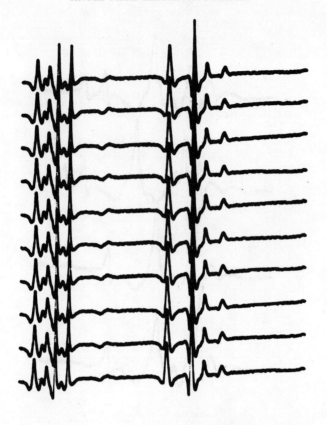

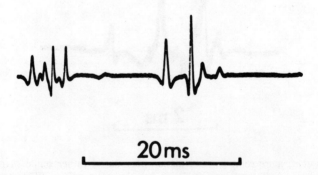

Fig. 20 Bizarre high frequency discharge in a patient with spinal tumour. 10 discharges
are superimposed below to show the constancy and low jitter of the complex.

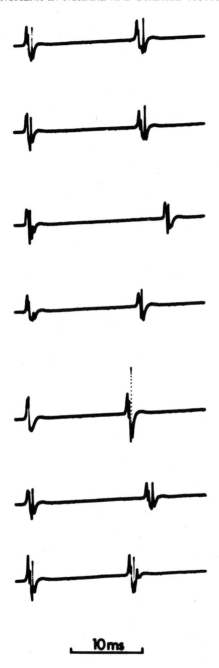

Fig. 21   Spontaneous discharges in a thenar muscle of a patient with carpal tunnel syndrome.
Notice double discharges of a triple potential with considerable jitter occurring at
moderately irregular rate.

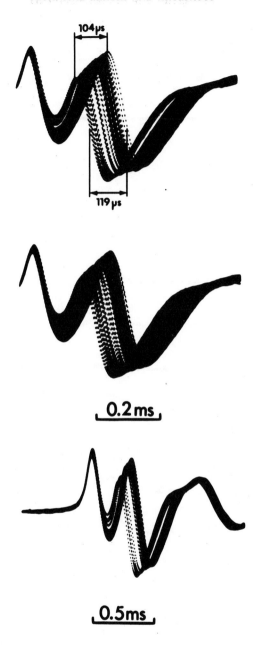

Fig. 22 Partial superimposition of the first two spikes. In manual measurement of the jitter, the range of interpotential intervals between the two peaks instead of the range of base line intersection points should be taken.

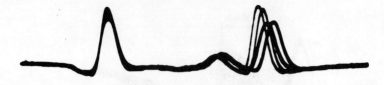

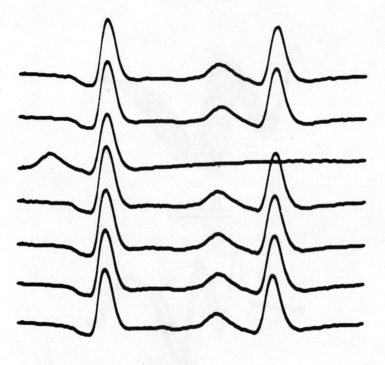

2 ms

Fig. 23   Tilting of action potential due to changing electrode position. Increased jitter and spurious blocking due to poor triggering.

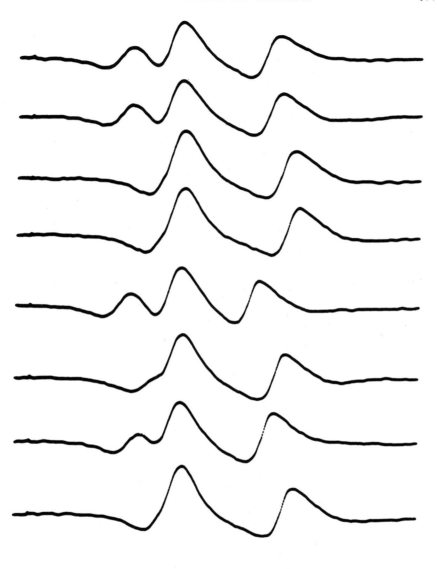

1ms

Fig. 24   Spurious disappearance of the first spike. The first spike occasionally merges with
         the second spike. (Bimodal jitter).

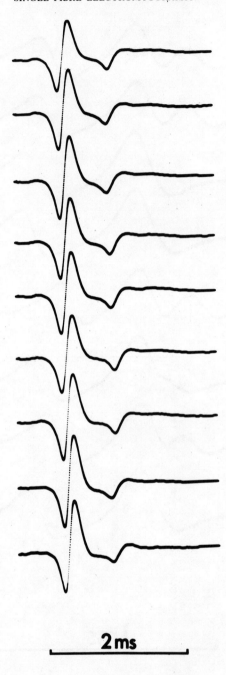

2 ms

Fig. 25   False double potential with low jitter. Probably slightly damaged muscle fibre.

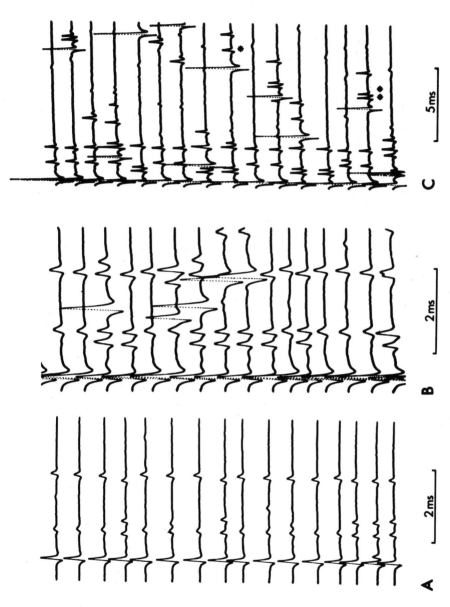

Fig. 26   Spurious blocking. The multiple potentials recorded in A belong to two different motor units, which is more clearly seen when the electrode position is slightly changed (B) and even better with slower sweep speed (C).

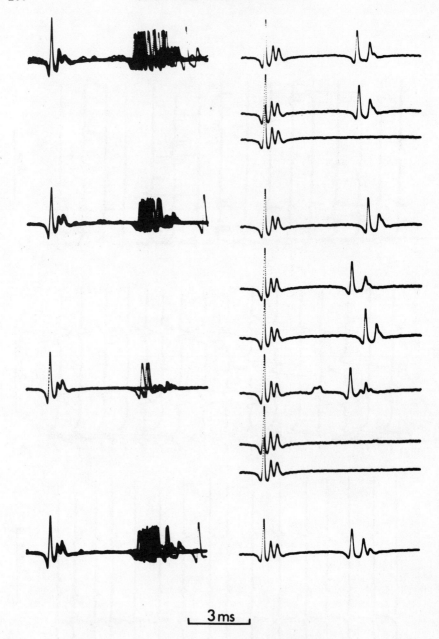

3 ms

Fig. 27 False neurogenic blocking. A triple potential followed by frequent extra-discharges that are recognized on superimposed recordings by the interval-dependent spike amplitude (lower at short intervals).

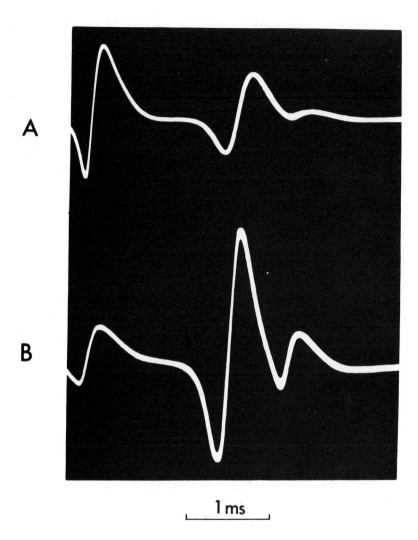

1 ms

Fig. 28   Error in estimating fibre density. Amplitude of first spike is made maximal in A and 2 fibres are counted. With slight change in electrode position a triple spike appears. However two of them are identical with those of the upper trace and this recording should not be counted. The electrode should be advanced far enough to lose all previously recorded fibres.

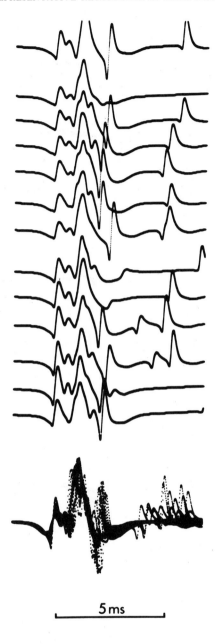

5 ms

Fig. 29   A complex potential in amyotrophic lateral sclerosis showing intermittent blocking
of 3 spike components and variable shape of the initial part of the complex.

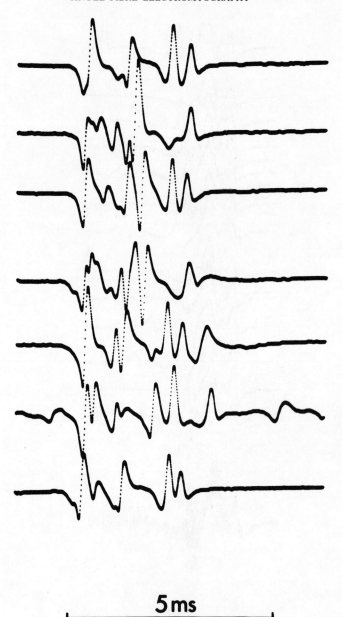

5 ms

Fig. 30   Recording from another patient with amyotrophic lateral sclerosis. The complex is variable in shape, at least two potentials block.

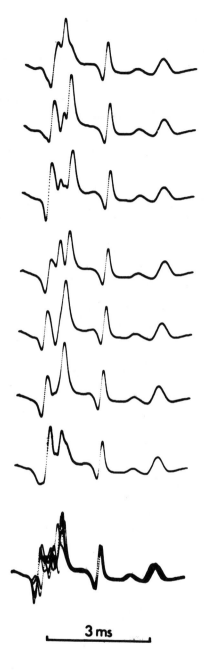

3 ms

Fig. 31 Another complex potential in amyotrophic lateral sclerosis showing variable initial part but stable later part.

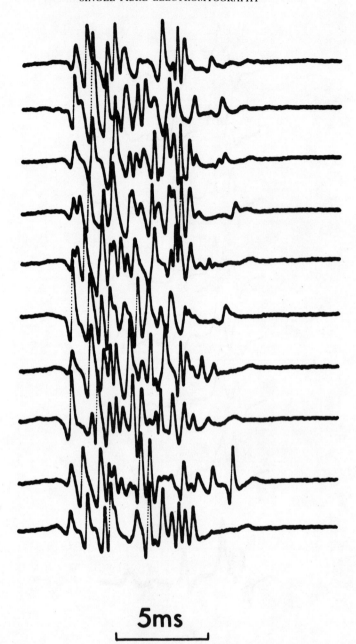

5ms

Fig. 32   Recording from extensor digitorum communis of a patient 15 years after poliomyelitis showing recent clinical deterioration.

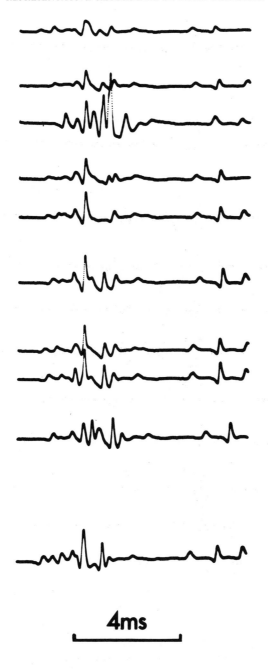

Fig. 33 A greatly variable complex potential in a patient with advanced juvenile spinal muscular atrophy.

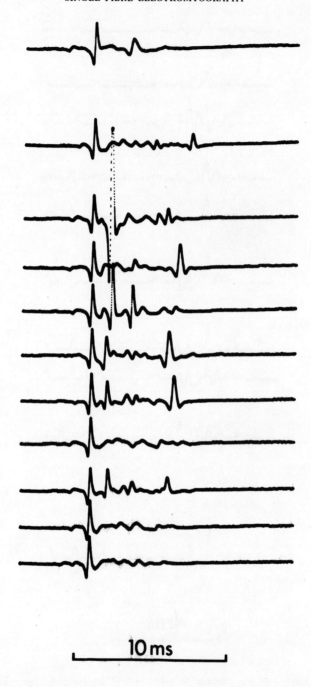

10 ms

Fig. 34   Another recording from the same patient as in Fig. 33.

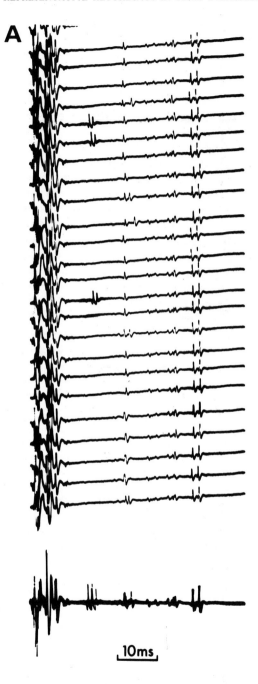

Fig. 35   Rather stable complex potentials with some single spike and concomitant blocking
        (A) from a patient with syringomyelia

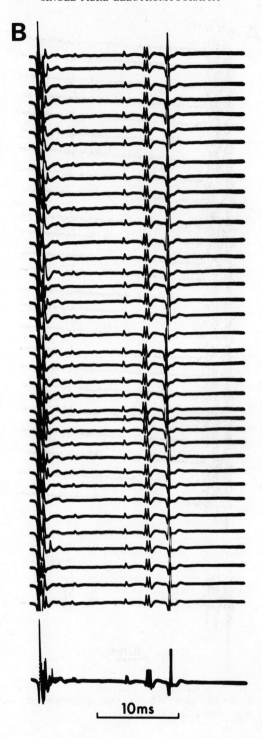

10ms

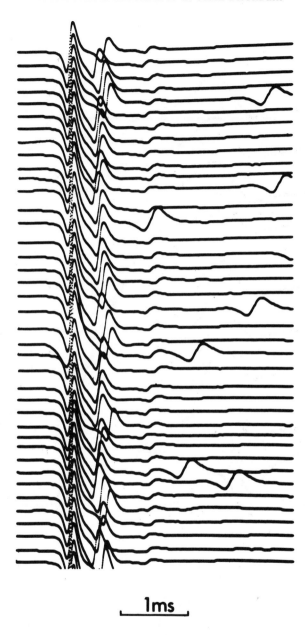

1ms

Fig. 36 A recording from four muscle fibres. Fibre No. 2 shows moderately increased jitter without blocking, fibre No. 3 shows practically normal jitter and fibre No. 4 has greatly increased jitter with frequent blocking. An example of non-homogeneous involvement of motor end-plates within one and the same motor unit in a patient with myasthenia gravis.

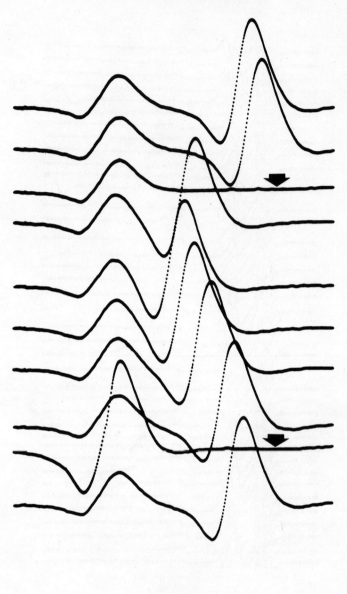

0.5ms

Fig. 37 A recording from a patient with myasthenia gravis showing large jitter and occasional blocking of either the first or the second potential (arrows).

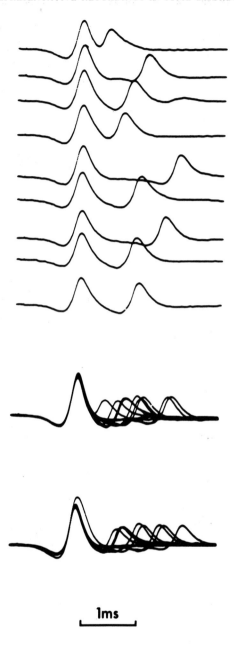

1ms

Fig. 38 A recording from a patient with myasthenia gravis with unusually large jitter without blocking. On the lower superimposed recording there is superimposition of both potentials in one trace.

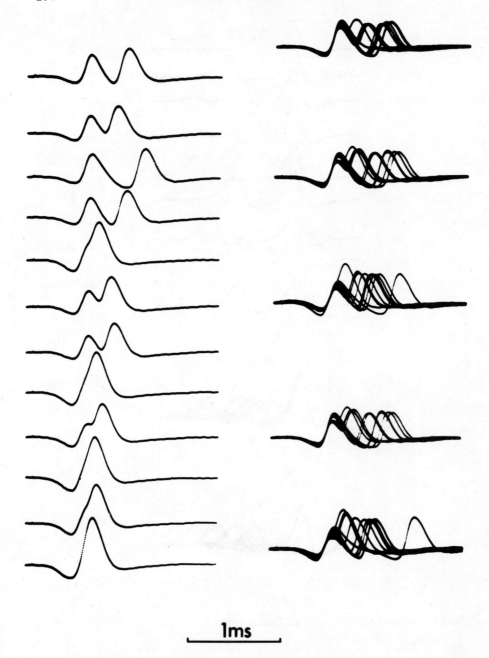

1ms

Fig. 39 A recording from a patient with myasthenia gravis. Large jitter with partial superimposition of the two potentials. Only 2% blocking.

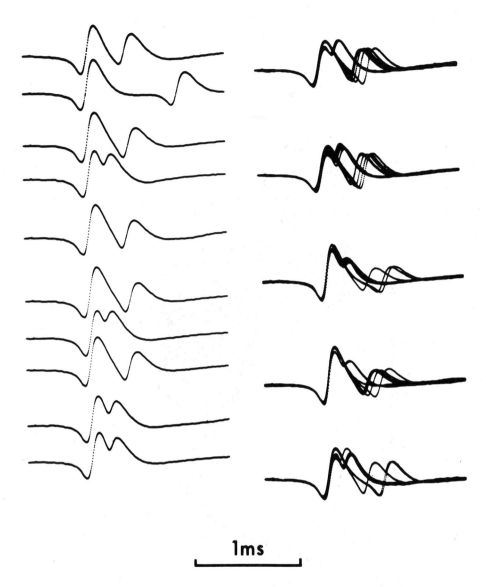

1ms

Fig. 40   Another patient with myasthenia gravis. The recording shows bimodal distribution
of interpotential intervals. The jitter in the early position is normal but in the late
position it is increased. In only one trace there is blocking.

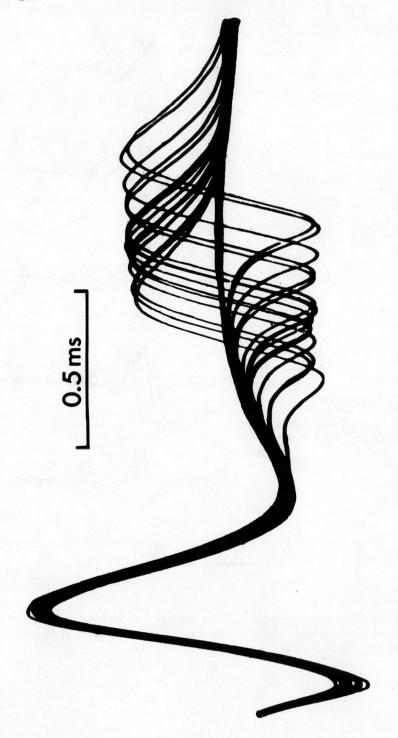

Fig. 41 Superimposed recording of a muscle fibre pair in mother of a boy with severe myasthenia gravis. About 30% of the recordings in this woman showed increased jitter, some of these without blocking.

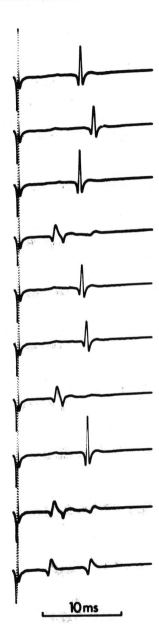

Fig. 42 A recording from a patient with tetany: spontaneous activity evoked by hyperventilation. Notice extra-discharges with variable amplitude, not quite clearly correlated to the interval to the extra-discharge in this case. When the extra-discharge
occurs at an interval below 5 ms the duration is very prolonged.

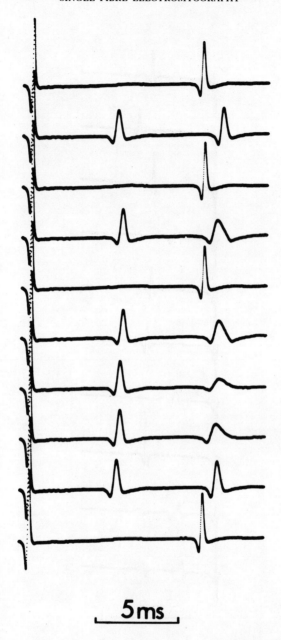

5ms

Fig. 43   Another patient with tetany. Doublets and triplets. The third potential (second extra-discharge) is very low and has very prolonged rise time.

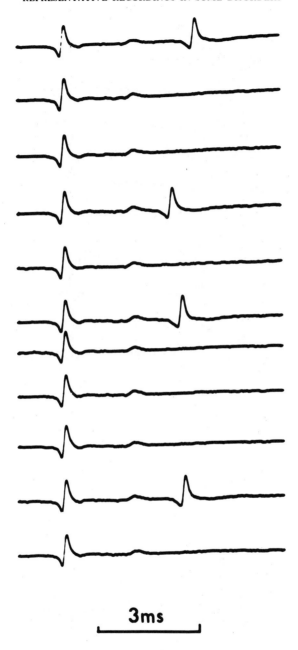

3ms

Fig. 44 A patient with myotonic dystrophy. Note long intervals and abnormal jitter with frequent blocking.

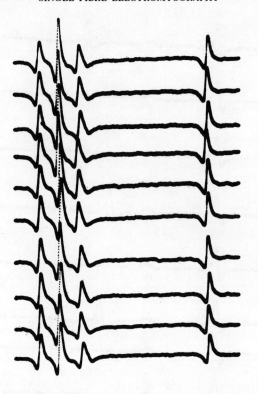

2.5 ms

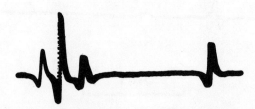

Fig. 45 A typical recording from a patient with Duchenne dystrophy showing moderately prolonged duration of the multiple potential with normal jitter.

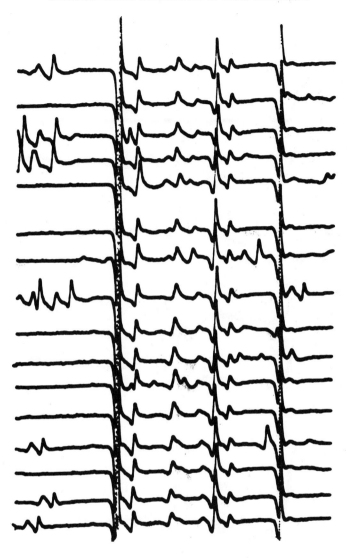

20ms

Fig. 46   Recordings from the EDC muscle of a 6-year-old boy with Duchenne dystrophy.

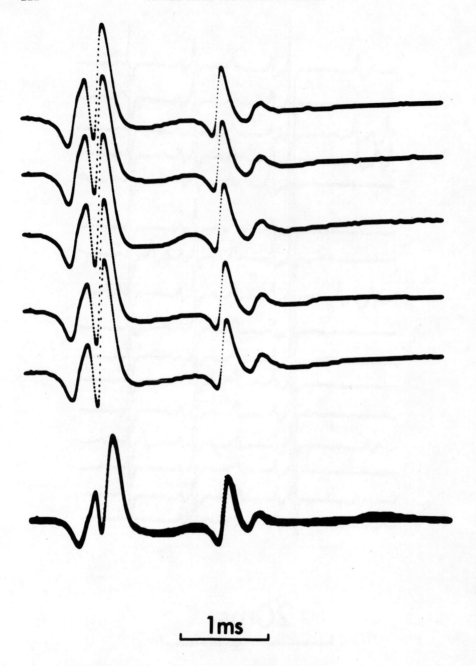

1ms

Fig. 47 A stable multiple potential (5 fibres) in a patient with chronic polymyositis in remission.

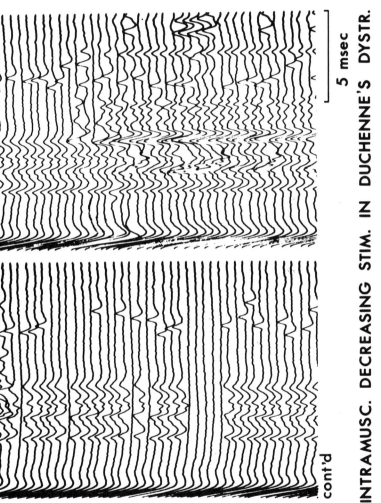

5 msec

cont'd

INTRAMUSC. DECREASING STIM. IN DUCHENNE'S DYSTR.

Fig. 48   Intramuscular (axonal) electrical stimulation in a patient with Duchenne dystrophy. On decreasing stimulus strength, there is simultaneous drop-out of several spikes at a time, indicating increased fibre density.

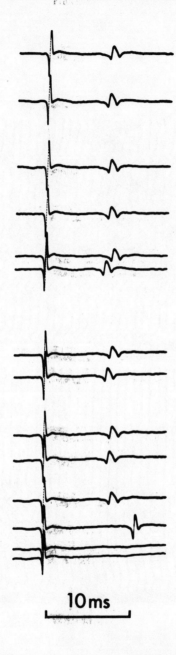

10 ms

Fig. 49   A patient with chronic polymyositis showing extra-discharges. These are both with short interval (7–11 ms) and longer intervals (40–60 ms) seen as shorter vertical distance and occurring especially after a short pause in activity.

SUBJECT INDEX

AUTHOR INDEX

GENERAL REFERENCES

ABERCOMBIE, M. and M.L. JOHNSON (1942): The outwandering of cells in tissue cultures of nerves undergoing wallerian degeneration. *J. Exp. Biol. 19*, 266–283.
ABERCOMBIE, M. and M.L. JOHNSON (1946): Quantitative histology of wallerian degeneration. Nuclear population in rabbit sciatic nerve. *J. Anat. 80*, 37–50.
ADLER, R.B., L.J. CHU and R.M. FANO (1960): Electromagnetic energy transmission and radiation. John Wiley. New York, London, Sydney.
ADRIAN, E.D. and D.V. BRONK (1929): Discharge of impulses in motor nerve fibres. *J. Physiol.* (Lond.) *67*, 119-151.
ANDREASSEN, S. and A. ROSENFALCK (1977): Recording from a single motor unit during strong effort. *Electroenceph. clin. Neurophysiol. 43*, 593.
BALLANTYNE, J.P. and S. HANSEN (1974): A new method for the estimation of the number of motor units in a muscle. 1. Control subjects and patients with myasthenia gravis. *J. Neurol. Neurosurg. Psychiat. 37*, 907–915.
BLOM, S. and J. RINGQVIST (1971): Neurophysiological findings in myasthenia gravis. Single muscle fibre activity in relation to muscular fatiguability and response to anticholinesterase. *Electroenceph. clin. Neurophysiol. 30*, 477–487.
BORENSTEIN, S. and J.E. DESMEDT (1975): Local cooling in myasthenia. *Arch. Neurol. 32*, 152–157.
BRANDSTATER, M.E. and E.H. LAMBERT (1969): A histochemical study of the spatial arrangement of muscle fibres in single motor units within rat tibialis anterior muscle. *Bull. Am. Assoc. Electromyogr. Electrodiagn. 82*, 15–16.
BROWN, W.F. (1972): A method for estimating the number of motor units in thenar muscles and the changes in motor unit counting with ageing. *J. Neurol. Neurosurg. Psychiat. 35*, 845–852.
BUCHTHAL, F., Ch. GULD and P. ROSENFALCK (1957): Multielectrode study of the territory of a motor unit. *Acta Physiol. Scand. 39*, 83–103.
BURKE, R.E., P. TSARIS, D.N. LEVINE, F.E. ZAJAC III and W.K. ENGEL (1973): Direct correlation of physiological and histochemical characteristics in motor units of cat triceps surae muscle. In: J.E. Desmedt (ed.), *New Developments in Electromyography and Clinical Neurophysiology.* Karger, Basel *1*, 23–30.
COËRS, C., N. TELERMAN-TOPPET and J.M. GERARD (1973): Terminal innervation ratio in neuromuscular disease. *Arch. Neurol. 29*, 215–222.
COËRS, C. and A.L. WOOLF (1959): The innervation of muscle. A biopsy study. Blackwell Scientific Publications, Oxford.
DESMEDT, J.E. and S. BORENSTEIN (1976): Regeneration in Duchenne-muscular dystrophy. Electromyographic evidence. *Arch. Neurol. 33*, 642–650.
DIAMANTOPOULOS, E and M.M. GASSEL (1965): Electrically induced monosynaptic reflexes in man. *J. Neurol, Neurosurg. Psychiat, 28* 496–502
DOYLE, A.M. and Rf. MAYER (1969): Studies of the motor units in the cat. *Cat. Bull. Sch. Med. Univ. Maryland. 54*, 11–17.
DUCHEN, L.W. and S.J. STRICH (1968): The effects of botulinum toxin on the pattern of innervation of skeletal muscle in the mouse. *J. Exp. Physiol. 53*, 84–89.

EDDS, M.V. (1950): Collateral reinnervation of residual motor axons in partially denervated muscles. *J. Exp. Zool. 113*, 517–552.

EDSTRÖM, L. and E. KUGELBERG (1968): Histochemical composition, distribution of fibres and fatiguability of single motor units. *J. Neurol. Neurosurg. Psychiat. 31*, 424–433.

EKSTEDT, J. (1964): Human single muscle fibre action potentials. *Acta Physiol. Scand.* 61 Suppl. *226*, 1–96.

ELMQVIST, D., W.W. HOFMANN, J. KUGELBERG and D.M. QUASTEL (1964): An electrophysiological investigation of neuromuscular transmission in myasthenia gravis. *J. Physiol. 174.* 417–434.

ENGEL, W.K. (1966): Histochemistry of neuromuscular diseases. Significance of muscle fibre types. Neuromuscular diseases. *2*, 67–101.

ENGEL, A.G., E.H. LAMBERT and T. SANTA (1973): Study of long-term anticholinesterase therapy. Effects on neuromuscular transmission and on motor end-plate fine structure. *Neurology 23*, 1273–1281.

ENGEL, A.G., B. MOKRI, F. JERUSALEM, H. SAKAKIBARA and O.B. PAULSON (1977): Ultrastructural clues in Duchenne dystrophy. In *Pathogenesis of Human Muscular Dystrophies.* L.P. Rowland (ed.), pp. 310–327.

ENGEL, A.G., M.TSUJIHATA, H. SAKAKIBARA, J.M. LINDSTROM and E.H. LAMBERT (1977): Ultrastructural evidence for acetylcholine receptor dysfunction in myasthenia gravis and its autoimmune model. In *Pathogenesis of Human Muscular Dystrophies.* L.P. Rowland (ed.), pp. 132–143. Excerpta Medica Amsterdam-Oxford.

FEINSTEIN, B., B. LINDEGÅRD, E. NYMAN and G. WOHLFART (1955): Morphologic studies of motor units in normal human muscles. *Acta Anat. 23*, 127–142.

FREUND, H.J., V. DIETZ, C.W. WITA and H. KAPP (1973): Discharge characteristics of single motor units in normal subjects and patients with supraspinal motor disturbances. In: J.E. Desmedt (ed.), *New Developments in Electromyography and Clinical Neurophysiology.* Karger, Basel *3*, 242-250.

FULLERTON, P.M. and R.W. GILLIAT (1965): Axon reflexes in human motor nerve fibres. *J. Neurol. Neurosurg. Psychiat. 28*, 1–11.

GOODGOLD, J. and A. EBERSTEIN (1972): Electrodiagnosis of neuromuscular diseases. Williams and Wilkins, Baltimore.

GRIMBY, L. and J. HANNERZ (1968): Recruitment order of motor units voluntary contraction: Changes induced by proprioceptive afferent activity. *J. Neurol. Neurosurg. Psychiat. 31*, 565-573.

GRIMBY, L. and J. HANNERZ (1976): Disturbances in voluntary recruitment order of low and high frequency motor units on blockades of proprioceptive afferent activity. *Acta Physiol. Scand., 29*, 207–216.

GRUENER (1977): In vitro membrane excitability of diseased human muscle. In *Pathogenesis of Muscular Dystrophies.* L.P. Rowland (ed.) pp. 242–258. Excerpta Medica Amsterdam-Oxford.

HAGBARTH, K-E. (1962): Posttetanic potentiation of the myotatic reflex in man. *J. Neurol. Neurosurg. Psychiat. 25*, 1–12.

HAKELIUS, L., B. NYSTRÖM and E. STÅLBERG (1975): Histochemical and neurophysiological studies of autotransplanted cat muscle. *Scand. J. Plast. Reconstr. Surg. 9*, 15-24.

HAKELIUS, L. and E. STÅLBERG (1974): Electromyographical studies of free autogenous muscle transplants in man. *Scand. J. Plast. Reconstr. Surg. 8*, 211-219.

HANNERZ. J. (1974): An electrode for recording single motor unit activity during strong muscle contraction. *Electroenceph. clin. Neurophysiol. 37*, 179-181.

HANNERZ, J. and L. GRIMBY (1973): Recruitment order of motor units in man: Significance of pre-existing state of facilitation. *J. Neurol. Neurosurg. Psychiat. 36*, 275-281.

HAYWARD, M. and R.G. WILLISON (1977): Automatic analysis of the electromyogram in patients with chronic partial denervation. *J. Neurol Sci. 33*, 415-423.

HAYWARD, M. (1977): Automatic analysis of the electromyogram in healthy subjects of different ages. *J. Neurol. Sci. 33*, 397-414.

HEILBRONN, E., C. MATTSON and E. STÅLBERG (1974): Immune response in rabbits to a cholinergic receptor protein: Possibly a model for myasthenia gravis. Excepta Medica Int. Congr. Series No 360. Recent Advances in Myology, *Proc. of the 3rd Int. Congr. on Muscle Diseases*, Newcastle Upon Tyne 15-21 Sept.

HEILBRONN, E., C. MATTSON, L-E. THORNELL, M. SJÖSTRÖM, E. STÅLBERG, P. HILTON-BROWN and D. ELMQVIST (1976): Experimental myasthenia in rabbits: Biochemical, immunological, electrophysiological and morphological aspects. *Annals of N.Y. Acad. Sci. 274*, 337–353.

HEILBRONN, E., and E. STÅLBERG (1978): The pathogenesis of Myasthenia Gravis. *J. Neurochem 31*, 5–11

HENNEMAN, E., G. SOMJEN and D.O. CARPENTER (1965): Functional significance of cell size in spinal motor neurones. *J. Neurophysiol. 28*, 560–589.

HENRIKSSON, K.G., O. NILSON, I. ROSEN and H. SCHILLER (1977): Clinical, neurophysiological and morphological findings in Eaton Lambert syndrome. *Acta Neurol. Scand. 56*, 117–140.

HOFFMAN, H. (1950): Local reinnervation in partially denervated muscle. *Austr. J. Exp. Biol. Med. Sci. 28*, 383–397.

HOPF, H.C. and A. STRUPPLER (1974): *Elektromyographie*. Thieme, Stuttgart.

HÅKANSSON, C.H. (1956): Conduction velocity and amplitude of the action potential as related to circumference in the isolated fibre of frog muscle. *Acta Physiol. Scand. 37*, 14-34.

HÅKANSSON, C.H. (1957): Action potentials recorded intra- and extra cellularly from the isolated frog muscle fibre in ringers solution and in air. *Acta Physiol. Scand. 41*, 190–216.

JENNEKENS, F.G.I., B.E. TOMLINSON and J.N. WALTON (1971): Data on the distribution of fibre types in five human limb muscles. *J. Neurol. Sci. 14*, 245-257.

KARPATI, G. and W.K. ENGEL (1968): Type grouping in skeletal muscle after experimental reinnervation. *Neurology* (Minneap.) *18*, 447-455.

KASHEF, R. (1966): A comparative and dimensional study of the node of Ranvier. Thesis, University of London.

KRNJEVIĆ, K. and R. MILEDI (1958): Motor units in the rat diaphragm. *J. Physiol.* (Lond.) *140*, 427-439.

KUGELBERG, E. (1973): Properties of the rat hind-limb motor units. In: J.E. Desmedt (ed.), *New Developments in Electromyography and Clinical Neurophysiology*. Karger, Basel *1*, 2-13.

KUGELBERG, E. and L. EDSTRÖM (1968): Differential histochemical effects of muscle contraction on phosphorylase and glycogen in various types of fibres: Relation to fatigue. *J. Neurol. Neurosurg. Psychiat. 31*, 415–423.

KUGELBERG, E., L. EDSTRÖM and M. ABRUZZESE (1970): Mapping of motor units in experimentally reinnervated rat muscle. *J. Neurol. Neurosurg. Psychiat. 33*, 319–329.

LENMAN, J.A.R. and A.E. RITCHIE (1977): *Clinical Electromyography.* Pitman Medical.

LICHT, S.: *Third edition of electrodiagnosis and electromyography.* Publisher: Licht E. 360 Fountain Street, New Haven, Connecticut.

LINDSTRÖM, L. (1970): *On the frequency spectrum of EMG signals.* Thesis. Res. Lab. Med. Electro. Gothenburg 1970.

LINDSTRÖM, L. (1973): A model describing the power spectrum of myoelectric signals. Part 1: Single fibre signal. *Technical Report 5.73.* Chalmers University, Gothenburg.

LUDIN, H-P. (1976): *Praktische electromyographie.* Ferdinand Enke Verlag, Stuttgart.

LUNDBERG, P.O., P.O. OSTERMAN and E. STÅLBERG (1969): Neuromuscular signs and symptoms in acromegaly. *Excerpta Medica Int. Congr. Series No 199. Muscle Diseases.* 531–534.

McCOMAS, A.J. (1977): *Neuromuscular Function and Disorders.* Butterworth and Co., London.

McCOMAS, A.J., P.R.W. FAWCETT, M.J. CAMPBELL and R.E.P. SICA (1971): Electrophysiological estimation of the number of motor units within a human muscle. *J. Neurol. Neurosurg. Psychiat. 34*, 121–131.

McCOMAS, A.J., R.E.P. SICA and M.J. CAMPBELL (1973): Number and sizes of human motor units in health and diseases. In: J.E. Desmedt (ed.), *New Developments in Electromyography and Clinical Neurophysiology.* Karger, Basel *1*, 55–63.

MILNER-BROWN, H.S., R.B. STEIN and R. YEMM (1973A): The contractile properties of human motor units during voluntary isometric contractions. *J. Physiol. 228*, 285–306.

MILNER-BROWN, H.S., R.B. STEIN and R. YEMM (1973B): Changes in firing rate of human motor units during linearly changing voluntary contractions. *J. Physiol. 230*, 371–390.

MILNER-BROWN, H.S., R.B. STEIN and R. YEMM (1973C): The orderly recruitment of human motor units during voluntary isometric contractions. *J. Physiol. 230*, 359–370.

MORRIS, C.J. (1969): Human skeletal muscle fibre type grouping and collateral reinnervation. *J. Neurol. Neurosurg. Psychiat. 32*, 440–444.

PETAJAN, J.H. and B.A. PHILIP (1969): Frequency control of motor unit action potentials. *Electroenceph. clin. Neurophysiol. 27*, 66–72.

ROBERTS, D.V. and S. THESLEFF (1969): Acetylcholine release from motor-nerve endings in rat treated with neostigmine. *Europ. J. Pharmacol. 6*, 281–285.

ROMANUL, F. and J. VAN DER MEULEN (1967): Slow and fast muscles after cross innervation. *Arch. Neurol. 17*, 387–402.

ROSENFALCK, P. (1969): *Intra and extracellular potential fields of active nerve and muscle fibres.* Akademisk Forlag 1-168, Copenhagen.

SANDERS, D.B., J.F. HOWARD and T.R. JOHNS (1978): Single fibre electromyography in myasthenia gravis. In press.

SCHWARTZ, M.S., A. MOOSA and V. DUBOWITZ (1977): Correlation of single fibre EMG and muscle histochemistry using an open biopsy recording technique. *J. Neurol. Sci. 31*, 369–378.

STÅLBERG, E. (1966): Propagation velocity in human muscle fibres in situ. *Acta Physiol. Scand.* 70 Suppl. *287*, 1–112.

THESLEFF, S. (1958): A study of the interaction between neuromuscular blocking agents and acetylcholine in the mammalian motor end-plate. *Acta anaesth. Scand. 2*, 69–79.

THESLEFF, S. (1977): Electrogenic properties of denervated mammalian skeletal muscle. In *Pathogenesis of Human Muscular Dystrophies.* L.P. Rowland (ed.) pp. 155–160. Excerpta Medica Amsterdam-Oxford.

THIELE, B. and A. BOEHLE (1975): Number of single muscle fibre action potentials contributing to the motor unit potential. *Fifth International Congress of Electromyography.* Rochester, Minnesota, U.S.A. Sept. 21–24, 1975.

TOKIZANE, T. and H. SHIMAZU (1964): Functional differentiation of human skeletal muscle. Univ. Tokyo Press. 1–62.

TRONTELJ, M. and J.V. TRONTELJ (1973): First component of human blink reflex studied on single facial motor neurones. *Brain Research 53*, 214–217.

VAN HARREVELD, A. (1945): Reinnervation of denervated muscle fibres by adjacent functioning motor units. *Am. J. Physiol. 144*, 477–493.

WARMOLTS, J.R. and W.K. ENGEL (1973): Correlation of motor unit behaviour with histochemical myofibre type in humans by open biopsy electromyography. In: J.E. Desmedt (ed.), *New Developments in Electromyography and Clinical Neurophysiology.* Karger, Basel *1*, 35–40.

WARSZAWSKI, M., N. TELERMAN-TOPPET, J. DURDU, G.L.A. GRAFF and C. COËRS (1975): The early stages of neuromuscular regeneration after crushing the sciatic nerve in the rat. Electrophysiological and histological study. *J. Neurol. Sci. 24*, 21–32.

WILLIAMSSON, E. and M.H. BROOKE (1972): Myokymia and the motor unit. *Acta Physiol. Scand. 26*, 11–16.

WOHLFART, G. (1958): Collateral regeneration in partially denervated muscles. *Neurology* (Minneap.) *8*, 175–180.

WRAY, S.H. (1969): Innervation ratios for large and small limb muscles in the baboon. *J. Comp. Neurol. 137*, 227–250.

SINGLE FIBRE EMG REFERENCES

1 ACHARI, A.N., J.V. TRONTELJ and R.J. CAMPOS (1976): Multiple sclerosis and myasthenia gravis. A case report with single fibre EMG. *Neurology 26*, 544–546.

2 BLOM, S. and J. RINGQVIST (1971): Neurophysiological findings in myasthenia gravis. Single muscle fibre activity in relation to muscular fatiguability and response to anticholinesterase. *Electroenceph. clin. Neurophysiol. 30*, 477–487.

3 BORENSTEIN, S. and J.E. DESMEDT (1975): Local cooling in myasthenia. *Arch. Neurol. 32*, 152–157.

4 CZEKAJEWSKI, J., J. EKSTEDT and E. STÅLBERG (1969): Oscilloscopic recording of muscle fibre action potentials. The window trigger and the delay unit. *Electroenceph. clin. Neurophysiol. 27*, 536–539.

5 CRAYTON, J., E. STÅLBERG and P. HILTON-BROWN (1977): The motor unit in psychotic patients. A single fibre EMG study. *J. Neurol. Neurosurg. Psychiat. 40*, 455–463.

6 DAHLBÄCK, L.O., J. EKSTEDT and E. STÅLBERG (1970): Ischemic effects on impulse transmission to muscle fibres in man. *Electroenceph. clin. Neurophysiol. 29*, 579–591.

7 EKSTEDT, J. (1964): Human single muscle fibre action potentials. *Acta Physiol. Scand. 61 Suppl. 226*, 1–96.

8 EKSTEDT, J., P. HÄGGQVIST and E. STÅLBERG (1969): The construction of needle multi-electrodes for single fibre electromyography. *Electroenceph. clin. Neurophysiol. 27*, 540–543.

9 EKSTEDT, J., B. LINDHOLM, S. LJUNGGREN and E. STÅLBERG (1971): The jittermeter: A variability calculator for use in single fibre EMG. *Electroenceph. clin. Neurophysiol. 30*, 154–158.

10 EKSTEDT, J., G. NILSSON and E. STÅLBERG (1974): Calculation of the electromyographic jitter. *J. Neurol. Neurosurg. Psychiat. 37*, 526–539.

11 EKSTEDT, J. and E. STÅLBERG (1963): A method of recording extracellular action potentials of single muscle fibres and measuring their propagation velocity in voluntarily activated human muscle. *Bull. Amer. Ass. EMG Electrodiagn. 10*, 16.

12 EKSTEDT, J. and E. STÅLBERG (1967): Myasthenia gravis. Diagnostic aspects by a new electrophysiological method. *Opuscula medica. 12*, 73–76.

13 EKSTEDT, J. and E. STÅLBERG (1969): Abnormal connection between skeletal muscle fibres. *Electroenceph. clin. Neurophysiol. 27*, 607–609.

14 EKSTEDT, J. and E. STÅLBERG (1969): The effect of non-paralytic doses of D-tubocurarine on individual motor end-plated in man, studied with a new electrophysiological method. *Electroenceph. clin. Neurophysiol. 27*, 557–562.

15 EKSTEDT, J. and E. STÅLBERG (1970): Electronic time interval measurements, data logging on magnetic tape and computer data analysis in single fibre electromyography. *Computer programs in Biomedicine 1*, 119–133.

16 EKSTEDT, J. and E. STÅLBERG (1973a): How the size of the needle electrode leading-off surface influences the shape of the single muscle fibre action potential in electromyography. *Computer Programs in Biomedicine 3*, 204–242.

17 EKSTEDT, J. and E. STÅLBERG (1973b): Single fibre EMG for the study of the microphysiology of the human muscle. In: J.E. Desmedt (ed.), *New Developments in Electromyography and Clinical Neurophysiology*. Karger, Basel *1*, 89–112.

18 EKSTEDT, J. and E. STÅLBERG (1975): Single muscle fibre electromyography in myasthenia gravis. In: K. KUNZE, J.E. DESMEDT (eds) *Studies in neuromuscular diseases.* Karger, Basel 157–161.

19 EKSTEDT, J., E. STÅLBERG and A-M. THORN-ALQUIST (1971): Impulse transmission to muscle fibres during intravenous regional anasthesia in man. *Acta anaesthes. Scandinav. 15*, 1–21.

20 FRIDEN, H. and E. STÅLBERG (1976): The sweller-selective gain control along the oscilloscope sweep. *Medical and Biological Engineering.* 697–698.

21 GATH, I. and E. STÅLBERG (1975): Frequency and time domain characteristics of single muscle fibre action potential. *Electroenceph. clin. Neurophysiol. 39*, 371–376.

22 GATH, I. and E. STÅLBERG (1976): Techniques for improving the selectivity of electromyographic recordings. *IEEE Transactions on Biomedical Engineering.* BME 23, No 6.

23 GATH, I. and E. STÅLBERG (1978): On the volume conduction in human skeletal muscle: In situ measurements. *Electroenceph. clin. Neurophysiol 43*, 106–110

24 GATH, I. and E. STÅLBERG (1978): The calculated radial decline of the extra-cellular action potential compared with in situ measurements in the human brachial biceps. *Electroenceph. clin, Neurophysiol 44*, 547–552

25 HAKELIUS, L. and E. STÅLBERG (1974): Electromyographical studies of free autogenous muscle transplants in man. *Scand. J. Plast. Reconstr. Surg. 8*, 211–219.

26 HENRIKSSON, K.G., O. NILSON, I. ROSEN and H. SCHILLER (1977): Clinical, neurophysiological and morphological findings in Eaton-Lambert syndrome. *Acta Neurol. Scand. 56*, 117–140.

27 HENRIKSSON, K.G. and E. STÅLBERG (1978): The terminal innervation pattern in polymyositis: A histochemical and SFEMG study. *Muscle and Nerve, 1*, 3–13.

28 LINDSTRÖM, L. (1973): A model describing the power spectrum of myoelectric signals. Part 1: Single fibre signal. *Technical report* 5.73. Chalmers University, Gothenburg.

29 LUNDBERG, P.O., P.O. OSTERMAN and E. STÅLBERG (1969): Neuromuscular signs and symptoms in acromegaly. *Excerpta Medica International Congress Series No 199. Muscle Diseases.*

30 LUNDBERG, P.O., E. STÅLBERG and B. THIELE (1974): Paralysis periodica paramyotonica. A clinical and neurophysiological study. *J. Neurol. Sci. 21*, 309–321.

31 MIHELIN, M., J.K. TRONTELJ and J.V. TRONTELJ (1975): Automatic measurement of random interpotential intervals in single fibre EMG. *Int. J. Bio-Medical Computing 6*, 181–191.

32 SANDERS, D.B., J.F. HOWARD and T.R. JOHNS (1978): Single fibre electromyography in myasthenia gravis. In press.

33 SCHILLER, E. and STÅLBERG (1978): F responses studied with single fibre EMG in normal subjects and spastic patients. *J. Neurol, Neurosurg. Psychiat. 41*, 45–53

34 SCHILLER, H.H. and E. STÅLBERG (1978): Human botulism studied with single fibre electromyography. *Arch. Neurol. 35*, 346–349

35 SCHILLER, H.H., E. STÅLBERG and M.S. SCHWARTZ (1975): Regional curare for the reduction of the safety factor in human motor end-plates studied with single fibre electromyography. *J. Neurol Neurosurg. Psychiat. 38*, 805–809.

36 SCHWARTZ, M.S., A. MOOSA and V. DUBOWITZ (1977): Correlation of single fibre EMG and muscle histochemistry using an open biopsy recording technique. *J. Neurol. Sci. 31*, 369–378.

37 SCHWARTZ, M.S. and E. STÅLBERG (1975): Myasthenia gravis with features of the myasthenic syndrome. An investigation with electrophysiologic methods including single fibre electromyography. *Neurology 25*, 1, 80–84.

38 SCHWARTZ, M.S. and E. STÅLBERG (1975): Myasthenic syndrome studied with single fibre electromyography. *Arch. Neurol. 32*, 815–817.

39 SCHWARTZ, M.S. and E. STÅLBERG (1975): Single fibre electromyographic studies in myasthenia gravis with repetitive nerve stimulation. *J. Neurol. Neurosurg. Psychiat. 38*, 678–682.

40 SCHWARTZ, M.S., E. STÅLBERG, H.H. SCHILLER and B. THIELE (1976): The reinnervated motor unit in man. *J. Neurol. Sci. 27*, 303–312.

41 SCHWARTZ, M.S. and M. SWASH (1975): Scapuloperoneal atrophy with sensory involvement: Davidenkow's syndrome. *J. Neurol. Neurosurg. Psychiat. 38*, 1063–1067.

42. STÅLBERG, E. (1966): Propagation velocity in human muscle fibres in situ. *Acta Physiol. Scand. 70* Suppl. *287*, 1-112.

43 STÅLBERG, E. (1976): Single fibre electromyography for motor unit study in man. In: M. Shahani (ed.), *The Motor System — Neurophysiology and Muscle Mechanisms*, pp. 79–92. Elsevier Scientific Publishing Company. Amsterdam, Oxford, New York.

44 STÅLBERG, E. (1977): Electrogenesis in human dystrophic muscle. In *Pathogenesis of Human Muscular Dystrophies.* Proc. of 5th Internat. Conf. of the Muscular Dystrophy Ass. L.P. Rowland (ed.) pp. 570–587. Excerpta Medica Amsterdam-Oxford.

45 STÅLBERG, E. (1978): Neuromuscular transmission studied with single fibre EMG. Proceedings of the 14th Congress of the Scandinavian Society of Anaesthesiologists. *Acta anaesth. Scand.* Suppl 70.

46 STÅLBERG, E. and J. EKSTEDT (1973): Single fibre EMG and microphysiology of the motor unit in normal and diseased human muscle. In: J.E. Desmedt (ed.), *New Developments in Electromyography and Clinical Neurophysiology.* Karger, Basel. *1*, 113–129.

47 STÅLBERG, E., J. EKSTEDT and A. BROMAN (1971): The electromyographic jitter in normal human muscles. *Electroenceph. clin. Neurophysiol. 31*, 429–438.

48 STÅLBERG, E., J. EKSTEDT and A. BROMAN (1974): Neuromuscular transmission in myasthenia gravis studied with single fibre electromyography. *J. Neurol. Neurosurg. Psychiat. 37*, 540–547.

49 STÅLBERG, E. and I. GATH (1978): Measurements of the uptake area of small size electromyographic electrodes. In press.

50 STÅLBERG, E. and O. HANSSON (1973): Single fibre EMG in juvenile myasthenia gravis. *Neuropadiatric. 4*, 20–29.

51 STÅLBERG, E., P. HILTON-BROWN, B. KOLMODIN-HEDMAN, B. HOLMSTEDT and K.B. AUGUSTINSSON (1978): Effect of occupational exposure to organophosphorus insecticides on neuromuscular function. *Scand. J. Work Environs and Health. 4.*

52 STÅLBERG, E., H.H. SCHILLER and M.S. SCHWARTZ (1975): Safety factor in single human motor end-plates studied in vivo with single fibre electromyography. *J. Neurol. Neurosurg. Psychiat. 38*, 799–804.

53 STÅLBERG, E., M.S. SCHWARTZ, B. THIELE and H.H. SCHILLER (1976): The normal motor unit in man. *J. Neurol. Sci. 27*, 291–301.

54 STÅLBERG, E., M.S. SCHWARTZ and J.V. TRONTELJ (1975): Single fibre electromyography in various processes affecting the anterior horn cell. *J. Neurol. Sci. 24*, 403–415.

55 STÅLBERG, E. and B. THIELE (1972): Transmission block in terminal nerve twigs: A single fibre electromyographic finding in man. *J. Neurol. Neurosurg. Psychiat. 35*, 52–59.

56 STÅLBERG, E. and B. THIELE (1973): Discharge pattern of motor neurones in humans. In: J.E. Desmedt (ed.), *New Developments in Electromyography and Clinical Neurophysiology*. Karger, Basel. *3*, 234–241.

57 STÅLBERG, E. and B. THIELE (1975): Motor unit fibre density in the extensor digitorum communis muscle. *J. Neurol. Neurosurg. Psychiat. 38*, 874–880.

58 STÅLBERG, E., B. THIELE and P. HILTON-BROWN (1973): Effect of succinylcholine on single motor end-plates in man. *Acta anaesth. Scandinav. 17*, 108–118.

59 STÅLBERG, E. and J.V. TRONTELJ (1970): Demonstration of axon reflexes in human motor nerve fibres. *J. Neurol. Neurosurg. Psychiat. 33*, 571–579.

60 STÅLBERG, E., J.V. TRONTELJ and M. JANKO (1974): Single fibre EMG findings in muscular dystrophy. In *Structure and Function of Normal and Diseased Muscle and Peripheral Nerve*. I. Hausmanowa-Petrusewicz and H. Jedrzejowska (eds) Polish Medical Publishers, Warsaw 185–190.

61 STÅLBERG, E., J. TRONTELJ and M.S. SCHWARTZ (1976): Single muscle fibre recording of the jitter phenomenon in patients with myasthenia gravis and in members of their families. *Annals of N.Y. Acad. Sci. 274*, 189–262.

62 STÅLBERG, E., J.V. TRONTELJ and M. TRONTELJ (1973): The jitter of single human muscle fibre responses to the stimulation of the motor axon. *Electroenceph. clin. Neurophysiol. 34*, 818.

63 THIELE, B. and E. STÅLBERG (1974): The bimodal jitter: A single fibre electromyographic finding. *J. Neurol. Neurosurg. Psychiat. 37*, 403–411.

64 THIELE, B. and E. STÅLBERG (1975): Single fibre electromyography findings in polyneuropathies of different aetiology. *J. Neurol. Neurosurg. Psychiat. 38*, 881–889.

65 TRONTELJ, J.K., M. MIHELIN, I. PLETERŠEK and L. ANTONI (1977): Micro computer for single fibre EMG. *Proceedings of First Mediterranean Conference on Medical and Biological Engineering*. Sorento, pp. 2.1–2.4.

66 TRONTELJ, J.K. and J.V. TRONTELJ (1968): Two examples of preparation

of biological signals for computation on a computer of average transients. *Automation and Instrumentation,* Fast, Alberto Mondadori, Milano, pp. 469–477.

67 TRONTELJ, J.V. (1968): H-reflex of single motor neurones in man. *Nature 220,* 1043–1044.

68 TRONTELJ, J.V. (1969): Measurement of neuromuscular jitter combined with tensilon test: A new diagnostic method for myasthenia gravis. (In Slovene). *Zdrav. vestn. 38,* 85–89.

69 TRONTELJ, J.V. (1969): Latency variation of single motoneurones in the H-reflex. *Electroenceph. clin. Neurophysiol. 27,* 723.

70 TRONTELJ, J.V. (1970): Reflex facilitation and inhibition of single motor neurones in man. *Jugoslav. Physiol. Pharmacol.* Acta *6,* 119–124.

71 TRONTELJ, J.V. (1971): A study of reflex activity of single spinal motor neurones in man. *Thesis* (in Slovene), University of Ljubljana.

72 TRONTELJ, J.V. (1973a): A study of the F-response by single fibre electromyography. In: J.E. Desmedt (ed.), *New Developments in Electromyography and Clinical Neurophysiology.* Karger, Basel *3,* 318–322.

73 TRONTELJ, J.V. (1973b): A study of the H-reflex by single fibre EMG. *J. Neurol. Neurosurg. Psychiat. 36,* 951–959.

74 TRONTELJ, J.V. and M.R. DIMITRIJEVIČ (1976): Single neurone studies of spinal and brain stem reflexes. International symposium on human reflexes and motor disorders. Brussels 1976. *Abstracts of communications,* J.E. Desmedt (ed.), pp. 168–169.

75 TRONTELJ, J.V., M. JANKO, C. GODEC, S. RAKOVEC and M. TRONTELJ (1974): Electrical stimulation for urinary incontinence. *Urol. Int. 29,* 213–220.

76 TRONTELJ, J.V. and E. STÅLBERG (1977): Spontaneous activity within the motor unit. 9th International Congress of Electroencephalography and Clinical Neurophysiology, Amsterdam, 1977. Abstract in *Electroenceph. clin. Neurophysiol. 43,* 613–614.

77 TRONTELJ, J.V., E. STÅLBERG and M.R. DIMITRIJEVIČ (1978): Spinal and brain stem reflexes recorded from single motoneurones. In press.

78 TRONTELJ, J.V., E. STÅLBERG and M. JANKO (1975): Responses of human single denervated muscle fibres to electrical stimulation. Fifth International Congress of Electromyography. Rochester. Minn. U.S.A., *Abstracts of communications* p.69.

79 TRONTELJ, J.V., E. STÅLBERG, M. TRONTELJ, M. JANKO, I. TIVADAR and B. JEREB (1975): Heredity in myasthenia gravis. Evidence of subclinical disease in some families. (In Slovene), *Zdrav. vestn. 44,* 229–232.

80 TRONTELJ, J.V. and M. TRONTELJ (1973): F-responses of human facial muscles. A single motoneurone study. *J. Neurol. Sci. 20,* 211–222.

81 TRONTELJ, J.V., M. TRONTELJ and E. STÅLBERG (1973): The jitter of single human muscle fibre responses in certain reflexes. *Electroenceph. clin. Neurophysiol. 34,* 825.

82 TRONTELJ, M. (1973): Reflex arc of the first component of the human blink reflex. *Thesis* (In Slovene), University of Ljubljana.

83 TRONTELJ, M. and J.V. TRONTELJ (1973): First component of human blink reflex studied on single facial motor neurones. *Brain Research 53,* 214–217.

84 TRONTELJ, M. and J.V. TRONTELJ (1978): Reflex arc of the first component of the human blink reflex. *J. Neurol., Neurosurg. and Psychiat. 41,* 538–547.